Pregnancy, poverty and health care

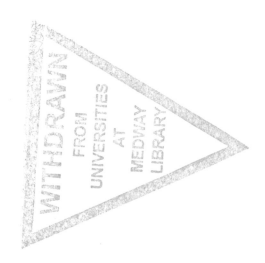

For my family, David, Ruth and Tom, who are my anchors in life's ocean. They have given me their unconditional love and support – each one in their individual and different way.

For Books for Midwives:

Senior Commissioning Editor: Mary Seager
Development Editor: Catharine Steers
Project Manager: Derek Robertson
Design: George Ajayi

Pregnancy, poverty and health care

Professor Sheila Hunt PhD, MBA, MScEcon, RGN, RM, ILTM
School of Nursing and Midwifery, University of Dundee, Scotland

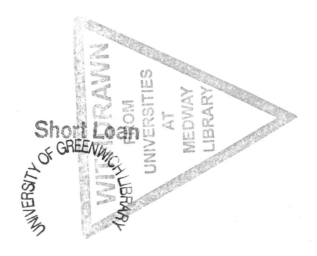

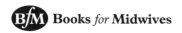 **Books** *for* **Midwives**

An Imprint of Elsevier Science

EDINBURGH LONDON NEW YORK OXFORD PHILADELPHIA
ST LOUIS SYDNEY TORONTO 2004

BOOKS FOR MIDWIVES
An imprint of Elsevier Limited

First published 2004

ISBN 0 7506 8798 3

British Library Cataloguing in Publication Data
A catalogue record for this book is available from the British Library

Library of Congress Cataloging in Publication Data
A catalog record for this book is available from the Library of Congress

The
publisher's
policy is to use
**paper manufactured
from sustainable forests**

Printed in China

Contents

Foreword

Jean Davis

There is a commitment on the part of the present Government to address issues of inequality with the aim of eradicating child poverty and the effects it has on health. Sheila Hunt has produced a very important book considering in depth the lives of some women with low incomes who are having children. The statistics stack up to indicate that the children born to poor women fare the worst in terms of morbidity and mortality. What this book does, however, is get behind the statistics to what is the only meaningful way of looking at how health and social care can begin to be effective; that is, with the individuals who collectively make up these figures.

The data were gathered using ethnographic research methods, using a combination of interviews and meeting women with low incomes who were using the maternity services. What emerges from the research is that there is no low income collective of women, but individuals raising children in a whole variety of ways, with an underlying hope that they are doing the job as best they can. Raising children anywhere is hard work, but within neighbourhoods where there is want, there is an even greater challenge. Part of this challenge for some of these women was to be treated with respect; respectability is an important concept but so difficult to achieve in the absence of adequate income. This book is essential reading for midwives and professionals working with pregnant women. It is a cautionary tale, in that it shows that not only do these workers have their own prejudices, but that these can and do undermine the women to whom the care is being given.

While doing the research, Sheila reflected and analysed her own beliefs and attitudes as an essential step in understanding her observations. If nothing else, this book challenges the reader to do likewise. In order to work effectively with individuals this must be a prerequisite, to avoid stereotyping and to offer sensitive, thoughtful and effective care. This is a tall order, but if midwives in particular are going to be 'with women' they have to be open to whom these women are, and what are their needs. They need to be willing to offer care unconditionally, without prejudice and fear. This is not easy.

It is not easy, either, to be working in environments that can be frightening; for instance, Sheila commented on being frightened of the dogs when she was visiting homes. Dogs are one thing, but the presence of dangers like drugs is another. What this book highlights is that however frightening this might be for the professional visitor, to actually live within a harsh environment is a constant challenge for women who are trying to do the best for their children.

Another form of inequality that is clearly a source of tension for some women, and no doubt for some men too, is that tension which exists between the sexes. A high proportion of the women in the study had experienced violence within their sexual partnerships. These relationships reflect a variety of forms, from accepting that having a partner, even a violent one, was better than being alone, to believing that independence, both financial and physical, was preferable. The study was undertaken in one area of the West Midlands, England, but I was struck by how similar the coping strategies and rationalisations about the various forms of inequality were to those seen in the 1980s in the Newcastle Community Midwifery Care Project. In that project, women in two neighbourhoods identified by low income levels were offered enhanced midwifery. The divide between the sexes was similar, as was the humour and common sense of so many of the women in the face of considerable hardship.

What readers should get from the book is that this common sense, or woman's intuition, needs to be given credence, and the humour heard. This takes time, effort and some humility. Answers do not all reside within professional expertise, not least because the right questions are not always asked. Above all else, this book shows that if inroads are going to be made into the detrimental effects of poverty on women and their children, it is essential to start from the individual woman's perspective. There can be no other starting place; midwives and others must have the courage to acknowledge that women's starting place is not always the same as that of the professionals. A change in beliefs, in attitudes and behaviour will not occur through imposition, but through co-operation and understanding – in current parlance, through partnership.

I feel very honoured to have been asked to write this Foreword; this book makes a crucial contribution to the efforts being made to eradicate the effects of poverty.

Jean Davies RN RM MSc
Midwife (and grandmother) who worked with women on low incomes

Preface

This book is about childbearing women who live in material poverty, and is based on research carried out in the West Midlands, UK, at the end of the twentieth century. The women who contributed to the research were all white and aged between 15 and 38. I did not work with women from black or ethnic communities; this was not by choice or design, it was simply an issue of access. Although the area had a high proportion of women from black and ethnic minority communities it proved impossible to gain access to those communities. The research sample was serendipitous; they were simply the women who agreed to give me their time and they were there when I was there.

The research then is a close and detailed examination of some aspects of their lives, but the issues that I explore are as much a reflection of my own agenda as anything else. I brought to the research nothing less than my life experiences, my background, my values and my beliefs. These own experiences have to some extent dictated what I saw, my own reflections and the questions I asked. These beliefs inevitably dictated the lines of enquiry, the areas that I studied in greater depth and to some extent the areas I chose not to follow.

It is generally acknowledged that disadvantage, in this case poverty, is socially constructed. Hence the 'knowledge' that I have created about this group of childbearing women living in poverty is itself part of a process of social construction. Wider and constantly changing social, economic and political forces affect women's experiences of childbearing and poverty; as a midwife and an author I was constantly torn between the issues of structures and the individual. In the end I conceded that that it is necessary to take both into account.

This book therefore is not only an analysis of structures, of social policy and an examination of the impacts of poverty on groups of people but it is also a detailed insight into the issues for individual women. In this book I debate the concept of poverty; I consider poverty as a woman's issue yet I am constantly drawn back to the individual. My role was to listen, to interpret and explain. I tried to stand back from the data, analyse it systematically and carefully, but I could not totally disengage from my own beliefs and experiences. I set out some of my own personal history in chapter one to share some of the issues that guided the research.

Throughout the research I was aware that I was seeing individuals coping, surviving, making some sort of sense of their experiences whilst they lived in material poverty. Some experienced prejudice and some had midwifery care that was dictated and influenced by their external appearance or their postal address. I found that to understand the experiences of this group of women I had to take into account both structures and individual agency. My aim throughout was to provide some insights for practising midwives so as to improve care. Uncovering these insights takes time, more time than the average midwife has at her disposal. Today midwives must draw on the major epidemiological studies that demonstrate the link between poverty and ill health; they must be aware of the links between social class and infant mortality rates. As midwives they will be all too familiar with the structural aspects of poverty, but they can also benefit from small-scale but in-depth research such as this that demonstrates that individual women experience childbearing and poverty in very different and individual ways. Only by studying both the structural aspects and the individual agency, the big picture and the finer detail, can we offer women the type of care they deserve. Midwives no longer need to be in power battles with either doctors or the women in their care. It really is time to accept that some women live lives that are different and challenging.

Midwifery has been part of the hierarchical and essentially paternalistic health-care system for over 100 years. Most midwives have been brought up to believe that is an important part of the role of the 'superior' health professional to help those sometimes 'inferior' individuals who get themselves into all kinds of difficulties. This book challenges each midwife to take responsibility for her own judgements and prejudices. There has to be a shift of focus away from routine care and onto the individual, especially when that individual fails to conform to the acceptable role and behaviour of women. It is no longer sufficient or acceptable to pronounce that poverty is the fault of the poor or to believe that there are simple solutions to complex problems. My feelings at the end of the research were that we have to tackle the intrinsic and mistaken beliefs that women alone can solve all their problems. If women were to simply 'stop smoking', 'leave their abusive partner', 'spend their money more wisely', 'avoid getting pregnant without a means of financial support', and of course 'attend clinics when requested' then all their problems would disappear and by implication midwives would have an obedient and conforming clientele.

This book presents midwives with a major challenge. It is no longer enough to give out advice and then despair at those who appear to fail to act upon that advice. If care is to significantly improve, midwives (like any successful business) must 'sell' what their 'customers' want to buy. This study sets out clearly what one group of women really want from the midwifery profession. Midwives have to see the individual beyond the statistics and they must take time to 'listen to women'. There must be a real willingness to engage with women, to take time to make human contact. Midwives must show that they are willing to look beyond structures, postcodes and stereotypes and see even if just for a moment the person behind the statistics. There is a need to rediscover the energy and potential of the Tracey, Mel and Sharon and work with them and the structures to make a difference.

Introducing the women

(To preserve anonymity, the names have all been changed.)

1. **Mel**: age 21, divorced. Three previous pregnancies, two live births, one miscarriage. Smokes. Experience of domestic violence in past year.
2. **Rachel**: age 22, cohabiting. Four previous pregnancies, three live births, one miscarriage. Smokes. Experience of domestic violence in previous year.
3. **Kelly**: age 20, divorced. No previous pregnancies. Smokes.
4. **Vicky**: age 21, single. Two previous pregnancies, one live birth, one miscarriage, one stillbirth. Smokes. Experience of domestic violence in past year.
5. **Jenny**: age 26, cohabiting. Six previous pregnancies, five live births, one miscarriage.
6. **Gerri**: age 24, married. One previous pregnancy, one abortion.
7. **Sally**: age 30, married. Four previous pregnancies, four live births. Smokes. Experience of domestic violence in previous year.
8. **Sarah**: age 15, single. No previous pregnancies. Experience of domestic violence in previous year.
9. **Sharon**: age 16, single. Smokes. Experience of domestic violence in previous year.
10. **Barbara**: age 36, married. Five pregnancies, three live births, one miscarriage. Smokes. Experience of domestic violence in previous year.
11. **Nikki**: age 17, married. Four previous pregnancies, four live births.
12. **Tracey**: age 29, cohabiting. Five previous pregnancies, five live births. Smokes.
13. **Tammy**: age 17, single. No previous pregnancies.
14. **Lisa**: age 20, single. One previous pregnancy, one live birth.
15. **Debbie**: age 19, single. Five previous pregnancies, three live births, one miscarriage, one abortion. Experience of domestic violence in previous year.
16. **Dawn**: age 36, divorced. Five previous pregnancies, five live births. Smokes. Experience of domestic violence in previous year.
17. **Judy**: age 30, divorced. Three previous pregnancies, two live births, one miscarriage. Smokes. Experience of domestic violence in previous year.

18. **Gaynor**: age 16, single. Three previous pregnancies. One live birth, two miscarriages. Smokes. Experience of domestic violence in previous year.
19. **Maria**: age 17, single. No previous pregnancies.
20. **Carol**: age 28, divorced. Three previous pregnancies. Three live births. Smokes. Experience of domestic violence in previous year.
21. **Kirsty**: age 23, single. Three previous pregnancies. Smokes.
22. **Joanna**: age 20, cohabiting. Two previous pregnancies, two live births.
23. **Hayley**: age 18, single. No previous pregnancies. Smokes.
24. **Claire**: age 38, divorced. Five previous pregnancies, three live births. Smokes. Experience of domestic violence in previous year.
25. **Emma**: age 15, single. Experience of domestic violence in previous year. Her first child, born when she was 13, had been adopted.

Introduction

Midwifery's unique opportunity

The beginning
Poverty: structural solutions
Midwives' unique contribution
Individualised care
Feminist poststructuralism: a way of
  seeing

Understanding social and policy
  discourses
No universal experiences, no universal
  solutions
Poverty: a woman's issue
Where next?

THE BEGINNING

This book is about individual women and their very individual experiences of childbirth and poverty in a West Midlands town at the end of the twentieth century. The book offers a challenge to midwives and other health-care professionals, it invites them to look beyond the statistics and the stereotypes and 'listen to women'. The purpose of the study, on which this book is based, was to determine the nature of the experience of pregnancy and poverty and to consider how some childbearing women make sense of their lives and experiences. The aim throughout the research was to understand the experience of childbirth from the perspective of women whose voices are seldom heard in official accounts, and who are unused to sharing their views or articulating their concerns and passions in a formal setting. By increasing knowledge and understanding, by sharing my insights and experiences of these women's lives, I will try to provide an accessible source of information for busy midwives. It takes time to 'listen to women'.

Many studies of women's experience of childbirth and official reports of women's views of maternity care, e.g. the 1998 Audit Commission report, have had to rely upon the views of white, literate, vocal, educated, usually older and articulate middle-class women, as these were the views that were readily available. There are exceptions to this rule (e.g. Gowridge *et al.* 1997, Graham 1984, Oakley 1992), but generally women living in poverty do not respond to official or formal information-gathering exercises. This study focuses on childbearing women who live in poverty, in order to articulate and attempt to understand some of the issues from their perspective. Therefore, through the book I hope to improve the understanding of these issues and, through that increased understanding, improve the care offered to women and enhance their experience of childbirth by teaching midwives how to recognise and understand the subjectivity of their own experience.

POVERTY: STRUCTURAL SOLUTIONS

In this book I will demonstrate how poverty still exists; it is difficult to define, difficult to measure, and equally difficult to find solutions. Government responses to poverty are by their nature structural. Policy responses have to address issues in public institutions, organisations, and public structures and systems. Government and public authorities look for 'big picture' solutions, so structural solutions tend to be ambitious with challenging targets and a clear focus on systems. The Social Exclusion Unit is a typical structural response as are the 'Sure Start' programmes and policy documents such as *Saving Lives: Our Healthier Nation* (Department of Health [DoH] 1999). These are structural responses to poverty and health inequality. Redistribution of wealth through income tax and benefits are also structural responses to poverty. In 1993 *Changing Childbirth* (DoH 1993) was another structural response to a maternity care system that was clearly failing to meet the needs of many women.

Whilst I believe that structural solutions are very important and I support the ways in which this government (Labour 1997-) is tackling inequality it seems to me that structural changes by their very nature inevitably do not always hit the mark. Structural changes are and will always be vitally important, but throughout this research it was very difficult to see the effects of major change or notice significant improvements in the lives of the women I met. This small group of women said that they briefly noticed a small increase in weekly child benefit payments but, for most part, their lives went on largely unchanged.

MIDWIVES' UNIQUE CONTRIBUTION

And so for this book: in the midst of structural change, health plans, targets and initiatives as well as energetic attempts to redistribute wealth there are individual women making their way through life, making ends meet, making sense of their lives and experiences. Midwives can work through the system; they can work with structural change at an individual level and make a real difference to women's lives and experiences of childbearing. Simply by seeing the individual, engaging with her agenda, listening carefully to her thoughts and fears we can change things for the better. Poststructuralism is a philosophy or a 'way of seeing': it looks beyond structures to individuals. I will return to this theme later in this chapter.

Childbearing women are living in poverty in the UK; they have individual needs and individual responses to childbirth and the maternity services. Midwives are in a unique position to work across the barriers and limitations of such structural responses and in so doing maximise the benefits and improve care to individual women. Midwifery by its very nature is individual; at some point in each woman's pregnancy career she will require the intervention of at least one midwife – there will be a meeting with one midwife and one woman. Midwifery care cannot be a group activity; at some stage it has to be delivered one to one. Here, by 'listening to women', the midwife has the unique opportunity to see the individual. As she listens she can look beyond the statistics, the published research evidence, the causes and effects, the analyses, and the 'big picture' solutions and (if only for a brief period) she can see the individual. She can listen, support, validate, advise, respect, ask sensitive questions and help each woman to embrace her childbirth experience and find her own solutions. She can listen to the woman and then ask her if she wants help to reduce her smoking habit. She can notice the absence of a fruit bowl and she can talk about her diet. She can listen sensitively, observe carefully and then ask if those abdominal bruises were really just an accident. I have discussed the complexity of this type of intervention in considerable detail in a book, *Pregnant Women, Violent Men* (Hunt and Martin 2001).

Midwives can use their unique position and relationship to listen, hear, notice and respond to women as individuals. Structural responses to poverty and inequality inevitably miss the individual and it is midwifery care that has the ability to counteract the 'misses' of structuralism's responses and help to get it right for individual women. This is the central message of this book.

INDIVIDUALISED CARE

The midwifery literature urges midwives to recognise the wants and needs of childbearing women and to treat them as individuals. This is a common and recurring theme in midwifery and yet it is not easily achieved. Lesley Page in her sensitive and visionary book *The New Midwifery* (2000) asks midwives to combine knowledge and clinical skills with science and sensitivity to provide successful midwifery practice. It is recognised that women have individual needs and yet it is often assumed that these wants and needs are the same for all women. These assumptions are most clearly set out in the government report *Changing Childbirth* (DoH 1993). I believe that this major report is incomplete. Of course the report was necessary and it has been of great importance in defining the quality of care that women deserve. There are clearly shared needs but there are also significant differences in women's needs; needs are often dictated by previous experiences, values and beliefs.

Providing individual care is not easy; in fact it is very difficult in an often overstretched service. It takes time to 'listen to women' and it requires a degree of insight and understanding to uncover the individual needs amidst the common needs. One of the problems with *Changing Childbirth* (DoH 1993) was that it assumed the needs of *all* childbearing women. This includes women who generally fail to respond to surveys and those who live in poverty on state benefits. The report assumed that there is a single, unified, childbearing woman's voice, which demands choice, control and continuity of care in the childbearing experience. For many women this is only the beginning and, for some, the least relevant part of their care.

Instinctively and based on my experience of midwifery, I knew that there was so much more to midwifery care. *Changing Childbirth* (DoH 1993) was the beginning, but individualised care needs more insight, more understanding, more thinking and listening. I knew that all women were different and I was always aware that many women still complain about their care. The report has certainly led to improvements in some aspects of the maternity services but I was convinced that there was still much more to do. There are other women having children, whose views were not heard and whose needs were under-represented. I was motivated to study this group of women because I felt that they, in common with other disadvantaged groups, suffered injustices not only because they were women but because they were poor and judged according to their social class.

Traditionally, studies of poverty are governed by the state structure that exists at the time and have tended to explore the impact of state policies used to counter the effects of poverty. This research is different; it uses ethnographic methods and a prolonged period of fieldwork to listen closely to the individual voices of women who are rarely heard. The book does not ignore state policy nor the impact of current social policy interventions, best described as Blair's 'Third Way'. It does not disregard the structural explanations of poverty nor the universal state-prescribed solutions but it concentrates on the impact of such policies, solutions and interventions on individuals. Through this close examination, I was able to uncover the intricate nature of individual women's experiences of pregnancy and poverty. I believe that by studying individuals in such depth and over an extended period of time, I was able to uncover the feelings, issues and concerns that were beneath the surface.

For the women I worked with, the structural changes demanded by *Changing Childbirth* (DoH 1993) of choice, control and continuity of carer were important concepts. However, the key issues for these childbearing women in poverty were much more complex. It was not the environmental issues like the wallpaper of the delivery room, nor the handing out of leaflets proclaiming 'choice' in childbirth. It was not the complex off-duty rotas for midwives, the teams and care schemes that sought to provide women with continuity of carer. It was much more than these structural and organisational concerns. The comprehensive changes since *Changing Childbirth* (DoH 1993) have significantly improved the care of many women but there are still complaints and many concerns. Individualised care may be Trust policy, it may be taught to student midwives in the classroom, but the reality is often different. To give women individual care is difficult. It requires much more than rhetoric and policies; it needs time, insight, intuition and considerable understanding. It also needs midwives to see the deficits and have the desire to do things differently. In this book I share some of my insights and experiences with the hope of improving care for childbearing women living in poverty. This study gave women the opportunity to talk about the issues that were important to them; it gave them the chance to participate in the setting of the health-care agenda, rather than merely being the recipients of policy changes. It gave them a chance to openly reject the rigid structures of organised health care and share those aspects of their lives that helped to form their experience of childbirth. For many women it provided a unique opportunity to be heard. Only by using ethnographic methods within a different 'way of seeing' (a poststructuralist feminist framework) was I able to see women as individuals, listen to what they had to say and examine what were the issues for them. Using this knowledge, I want to lead other midwives towards looking beyond the outward physical signs of poverty and addressing the needs of women as unique individuals undergoing the life-changing experience called motherhood. In the midst of structural change and strategic reviews of the maternity services, there must be a place for the needs of individual women to be heard.

The data in this research were collected using ethnographic methods and various themes emerged during the analysis. I have chosen to develop some themes and, of course, I have had to ignore others. The women in the study along with their own mothers, the grandmothers, had well-developed notions of responsibility, doing what was 'right' and a powerful need to protect and care for their children. This was often closely linked with the drive to be seen as respectable and accepted. These themes will be developed in subsequent chapters. I found that women's lives were complex, varied and sometimes very difficult; they willingly contributed to the research, gave me their time and shared their thoughts and feelings. They agreed that I could make tape recordings of their words and make notes about what I saw and thought.

FEMINIST POSTSTRUCTURALISM: A WAY OF SEEING

I began this research believing that I was a radical feminist; women were oppressed because they were women, society was patriarchal (dominated by men) and generally men as a group were defined as the main enemy. Women were frequently ruled by men and men generally exerted power over women. I was angry and felt that my mission was to expose such oppression and empower women in their struggle. But the reality of my research findings did not match my rhetoric and my preconceived theoretical framework or my explanation of my 'way of seeing'. Throughout this research, I was aware that I was studying a diverse group of women who had in common a life surviving on state benefits. I was aware of the government and health reports that made statements about health and poverty and I knew the conclusions that such reports made. I was drawn by the arguments that favoured the redistribution of wealth but felt that the rhetoric did not match the complexities of the lives of the women I was studying. Concluding that women simply 'need more money' ignores the subtle differences between individuals, and at this point I knew that the theoretical underpinning of my work had moved on from the anger of radical feminism. I found the solution to my dilemma in the theories described by Chris Weedon (2000) as 'feminist poststructuralism'. There is no simple definition of either feminism or poststructuralism. Beasley (1999) describes feminism as 'a troublesome term'. It is certainly complex, diverse and probably best described as a continuum from the most revolutionary in radical, Marxist/socialist and antiracist approaches, to those approaches influenced by poststructuralism/postmodernism. Feminist theory and feminisms are not a united movement, but in a very general sense they share an underlying concern for women and a desire to improve the lot of women. In this research I wanted to improve the lot of childbearing women living in poverty. I felt strongly that this group were doubly disadvantaged: disadvantaged by poverty and by being women in what often still felt like a male-dominated world. Feminism is based on a belief that there is something wrong with society's treatment of women in that women are systematically disadvantaged, even exploited. Some women pursue feminist goals but reject the feminist label, seeing it as elitist or racist and a form of political and cultural imperialism on the part of white women who are privileged in every way except for their gender (Bryson 1999). Feminist theory underwent a major transformation during the late 1980s and early 1990s. In particular, the assumption of 'difference' based on biology has been rejected. Similarly, the beliefs that universalised experience and the assumptions that women had more in common with other women as opposed to men have been rejected by those subscribing to a postmodern/poststructural view (Annandale 1998). Weedon describes feminism as:

'Politics directed at changing existing power relations between women and men in society. These power relations structure all areas of life, the family, education and welfare, the world of work and politics, culture and leisure. They determine who does what and for whom, what we are and what we might become' (Weedon 2000:1).

This study demonstrates the impact of some of the existing power relations between some men and some women. I found ample evidence of these power relations; they were evident between men and women but also between husbands, partners, boyfriends, and doctors' receptionists and midwives and other health professionals. Power is exerted in a range of settings: the home, the antenatal clinic, the GP clinic, and in women's homes. Midwives and other health professionals had no difficulty in knowing and expressing who was in charge.

Now a little more debate on this 'way of seeing' the world. Poststructuralism defies a simple definition; it was developed in France and the USA around a number of philosophers including Foucault, Kristeva, Derrida and Irigaray. Poststructuralists criticise the attempt to build grand theories; instead, they argue that we can only understand the world in partial, specific and local ways. In this study I have tried to understand something of the world of childbearing women at the end of the twentieth century. My understanding will inevitably be partial, specific to this group of women and local to the West Midlands, but there are common threads, common issues and experiences that can be used to increase our understanding of other childbearing women and their experiences. It would not be right to claim that my approach is the right one; the questions that I asked and the themes I developed reflected my own background and experiences. If the study were replicated, others would no doubt develop other themes, ask different questions and see other issues. There is no right answer, no certainty, but presented here is my interpretation of what I saw and heard.

For centuries philosophers have acknowledged that the world is fluid, changing, as well as inherently complex and fragmented. That has always been uncomfortable to traditional scientists, and the modernists at the turn of the twentieth century responded to that discomfort by assuming that there was a natural order followed by all societies that was cyclical, that could be discovered, described and understood. They believed that there existed a pre-prepared pattern of things that could be uncovered and described. Poststructuralists (and I now declare that I am one), however, accept that there is no definitive answer and that responses and reactions are determined largely by the individual. I reached this position after spending long periods 'listening to women'. I tried in vain to find definite answers, clear problems, causation and solutions but often failed. My neat data was not neat; there were inconsistencies, irregularities and inexplicable differences. Poststructuralists do not search for a definitive structure that will lend itself to social and political progress. The influence of the structure depends upon the nature of the individual; universal solutions cannot exist for there is not a universal response. In other words there is no simple solution to the 'problems' (as defined by society) of being pregnant and existing on state benefits. There are ample opportunities for midwives to see beyond the problems and see the unique issues for each woman. In each chapter of the book there is the opportunity to see the unique issues for each woman, and to begin to ask what can be gained when a midwife engages with, makes human contact with and relates on a different, perhaps even spiritual, level with the woman. To be 'with woman' is part of the rhetoric of midwifery. Now we should be thinking in terms of getting alongside her, to be with her and support her as she moves into society's most important role, that of parent and teacher to the next generation.

In an interesting example, I met one woman who had a previous history of a traumatic birth and surgical delivery of her baby. Despite being of a very small stature, anaemic, social class V, and single, she was determined to have a home birth. For her, the system had failed; in her previous pregnancy she had felt violated and totally out of control. She looked back on her experience with fear and anxiety. In this pregnancy she was determined to be in control of her childbirth experience. It took a very special community midwife to support her through a long labour at home and then escort to her hospital for another caesarean section. Woman, baby and midwife did well and did more than simply survive the experience. Her needs were unique to her and related to her own previous experiences. They were coloured by her relationship with her mother, with her feelings about the pregnancy and her relationship with the baby's father. Some women will share a difficult childbirth experience but each individual carries a unique combination of events that shapes not only their individual needs but also their whole being.

Poststructuralists attempt to find an understanding behind the apparent truths yet do not seek to replace one truth or theory with another. In this book I have tried to look beyond the obvious, the superficial and the expected explanations. By taking time, by listening carefully to women, over an extended period of time and hopefully without prejudice and preconceived notions of what is right and wrong, I have tried to describe the complexity of some of their truths. In the chapters that follow, this complexity will unfold.

Mary Hawkesworth (1989) explains feminist postmodernism (the terms poststructural and postmodern are often used interchangeably) in the following way:

'Feminist postmodernism rejects the very possibility of a truth about reality. ... They advocate a profound scepticism regarding universal (or universalising) claims about the existence, nature, and powers of reason ... they urge instead the development of a commitment to plurality and the play of difference' (1989:535).

Hence again we see that the nature of truth is particularly important: there is no truth, fact or theory that explains the meaning of pregnancy and poverty. In this book it will be seen that there are many explanations, many stories, many different voices, and many different ways in which women experience childbirth and poverty. There are many different ways in which individual women respond, react, and cope with their experiences; they all move onward in their lives making sense of experiences in different ways. To offer 'universal solutions' for their 'condition' is inappropriate and for the most part often irrelevant. The messages to women are clear; they are told: 'don't get pregnant [if you do not have a husband]'; 'eat a better diet'; 'attend antenatal classes'; 'go to the clinic'; 'have a scan'; 'breast-feed your baby'; 'leave your abusive partner' etc. As midwives we are generally more comfortable with universal solutions; we like checklists, we like simple responses, we have been taught the causes of most things and we know the effects so we are comfortable with lists, solutions, action plans. However, we can easily miss the individual who is not conforming to our plan and to pre-prescribed and often pat solutions. This book challenges us as midwives to avoid simple solutions and look beyond the obvious.

The central message is that life is complex, people's lives and experiences are complex, and there are no simple solutions. It also became clear that different life events could be ascribed different meanings by different observers. For me it was a disaster that a young boy was found lying in the street unconscious with a drug overdose. For his mother it was a relief; it meant that the local drug pushers would now go elsewhere. In this research, I brought my own history, biases, experiences and social class to search for meanings in aspects of women's lives. In the search for meanings, the meaning of an object, action or social institution is not inherent in it, but is called into being by words. There are no wrong meanings or 'true' meanings. Meaning is not fixed and waiting to be discovered but can be endlessly constructed and reconstructed through words, which have meanings in relation to other words. Weedon (2000:31) argues that 'we are neither authors of the way in which we understand our lives, nor are we unified rational beings'. It is through language that we are able to give meaning to the world and act to change it. In this study, I tape-recorded and transcribed the many different voices of the women in order to give meaning and to begin to understand something of the complexities of their lives.

Like most midwives, I have worked in the health service for most of my working life and I have been brought up on a diet of scientific research and the randomised controlled clinical trial. I have been taught that the 'truth' is out there and the solutions to the major problems of humanity will stem from finding the truth. Indeed much of the literature presented in this book is offered as a truth. For example, 'babies born to families in social class V are more likely to be low birth weight and more at risk of perinatal death'. However, some of these women had low birth-weight babies, but some did not; some women were smokers, but some were not; some breast-fed their babies, others did not. However, poststructuralist discourses reject the claim that scientific theories can give access to truth. Science can only ever produce specific, partial, incomplete knowledge. Much of the medical literature, which is used in this book, is written in such a way as to imply objectivity. The very style of language used can intimidate and imply assumptions of truth and validity. Bryson (1999) argues that our understanding of the lives of childbearing women living in poverty can never be complete; our knowledge is always limited and partial. This work, then, cannot claim to know the 'truth' about these women, but it can only add to our understanding of poverty and our understanding of some women's experiences of childbearing and poverty.

UNDERSTANDING SOCIAL AND POLICY DISCOURSES

To further this explanation and develop the argument or indeed the justification of poststructural feminism as a framework for the study, it is important to briefly consider the term *discourse*. Discourse is a term used by Foucault (and many others) and is described as the relationship between meaning, definitions, statements and the institutions and social networks that give them authority and validity. For example there is a policy discourse that argues that teenage pregnancy is a bad thing. Everyone believes it, the government is trying hard to stop it and it would probably be regarded as heresy to suggest that having a healthy baby at the peak of a woman's physical health was a good thing. Hence the policy discourse exists. It is a relationship between the meanings attached to the term 'teenage pregnancy', the definitions, and the statements that are made by government and others about it. It is a social and policy discourse, which informs the way we think, respond, act and plan. In this case it assumes a universal truth about the nature of pregnancy in teenage women. According to Hughes and Sharrock (1997:23) discourse is 'a complex structure governed by a system of rules which identifies the things that can be talked about, the things that can be said about them, which things can be said by which kinds of persons'. Ramazanoğlu (1993) offers a further explanation of Foucault's key term:

Discourses are:

'historically variable ways of specifying knowledge and truth. They function (especially in scientific discourses) as sets of rules, the operation of these rules specify what is and what is not the case' (1993:19).

Discourses are powerful and the power may be exercised by officials in institutions, midwives in maternity units, or in other practices. The teenage pregnancy discourse dictates policy, provision, attitudes, financial benefits and many more. To use another example: the *Changing Childbirth* report (DoH 1993) rhetoric insists that *all* women want and need choice, control and continuity of care in their childbirth experience. Policy and planning were informed by that discourse. Power is constituted in discourses and it is in those discourses, such as in clinical medicine and in social policy, that the power lies. Foucault (1980) argues that discourses produce truths and 'we cannot exercise power except through the production of truth'. Of course, not all discourses carry equal weight or power. There are dominant discourses, for example in social policy where women's place is seen in the home and dependent on the man whose role is the provider. There are also conflicting and contradictory discourses, for example those that urge women who are mothers of young children to move from 'welfare to work' and not be dependent on the state for support but at the same time stay at home to be good parents to their children. For the women in this study the dominant discourse of what constitutes 'normal family life' was also powerful. The so-called norms of heterosexuality, dependency on men and compulsory motherhood were powerful drivers for women. Later I will explore how, for some women, motherhood and an approved relationship with a man was a passport to respectability.

Beasley (1999) summarises poststructural thinking as stressing plurality rather than unity, rejecting the concept of women as a homogeneous category and refusing to acknowledge that there is such a thing as a universal experience. In this study, it was not possible to say that all of the women experienced poverty, childbirth, oppression or even domestic violence in the same way. Their experiences were unique and their responses individual. Poststructuralism theorists argue that there is no single structural or underlying explanation but there are multiple determinants. Poststructuralists, according to Beasley (1999:91), 'tend to stress the shifting, fragmented complexity of meaning (and relatedly of power), rather than a notion of its centralised order'.

Searching for meaning, then, is ongoing; meaning is neither entirely arbitrary nor absolute or eternal. We know what we know now, but even as it is written, so it changes. Meaning can be endlessly constructed and reconstructed through words, which have meanings in relation to other words. In the same way, understanding can never be final or complete and knowledge is always only partial and limited.

NO UNIVERSAL EXPERIENCES, NO UNIVERSAL SOLUTIONS

Bryson (1999) argues that there is no universal experience, no normalising account, no woman's voice, no single cause and no universal experience of oppression. In the same vein, there is no single solution to the 'woman problem'; instead, she argues that there are multiple determinants. The poststructural feminists refuse to sanctify a persecuted feminine identity shared by all women. It was clear from the evidence of this study that not all women are oppressed; they were not hapless victims but some had the power to change aspects of their lives.

In this book, I support these ideas and beliefs and recognise that the findings of this research will not apply to all women, or to all childbearing women living in poverty. Not all women who live in poverty with children will share the same experiences. In searching for meaning, it is recognised that there is no universal truth but another step along the way of understanding something of what is being seen. There are multiple ways of being a woman, multiple ways or paths of resistance but some common themes in the experience of being pregnant and living on state benefits. This research rejects the notion of universalised and normalising accounts of women as a group. It does not claim to represent or describe the experience of all childbearing women living in poverty. Not all women live in poverty, have children and share the experiences of this group of women and not all women are oppressed and abused. The women who contributed to this study were all very different, they had different ideas, values and experiences; however, they did share some common experiences, many struggled with poverty and the demands of small children, and over half of the sample had been subjected to physical and psychological abuse from their partners during their pregnancy. Many were driven by a need to be seen as respectable and all had a strong sense of responsibility for their children. In undertaking this research I believed that their accounts of their experiences were important and the search for meaning worthwhile.

POVERTY: A WOMAN'S ISSUE

In this book, I will try to explain how poverty is a far more significant issue for women, especially childbearing women, than for the men in their lives. However, first it is necessary to define poverty as a concept and explore the theoretical explanations of poverty. In later chapters, I will demonstrate how the consequences of poverty are greater, and the struggle to cope with poverty is more of an issue, for some women than it is for some men. In the confusing and complex world of objectivity and subjectivity it is possible to conclude that there are universal effects of poverty and these effects impact on women in ways that are different to men. This issue is discussed in greater detail in the next chapter.

In the UK, there are considerably more women in poverty than men. Access to the labour market is severely limited by dependent children. According to the Office of National Statistics (ONS), 59 per cent of adults supported by income support are women. The government defines the poor as 'those who have a disposable income of less than half the average equivalent disposable income per capita'. One third of households are currently in receipt of means-tested benefits and the number of pregnant women on means-tested benefits is now one in three. In Britain, 14 million people live on half the average income and one in three children live in poverty (*Family Resources Survey*, ONS 1996/97). As the structure of the typical household has changed, with increases in divorce and cohabitation, the proportion of families headed by a lone parent has increased; the net result is that women are more independent of men, but poorer.

In the UK, the 1990s have seen unprecedented economic and social change; there has been a major collapse in the manufacturing industry with the share of employment reduced from 32 per cent in 1973, to 25 per cent in 1983, and to 19 per cent in 1993. This represents a decline from 7.8 to 4.6 million people working in the manufacturing industries (OPCS 1995b). According to *Social Trends 28*, 35 per cent of men and 22 per cent of women were employed in the manufacturing industries in 1978, but in 1997 the number of men had reduced to 26 per cent and women to 10 per cent (ONS 1998b). According to the Office of Population Censuses and Surveys (OPCS), the trends suggest a further fall in the manufacturing share of employment and a corresponding rise in the numbers of those who work in the service sector. These changes have had a major impact on the structure and nature of social life in Britain. The significance of social class and economic inequality is still seen in relation to inequalities in health. Navarro (1994) argues that class divisions are as entrenched as ever they were, and the possibility of class action remains despite, or perhaps because of, the major changes in the nature of employment. The manual/non-manual divide is outdated, as is the definition of the single middle class. Rose and O'Reilly's (1998) work, on behalf of the government, on the reconstruction of classes (in particular for use in the 2001 census) is discussed later, but class still exerts a powerful force on society even though the nature and form of class have changed considerably.

WHERE NEXT?

So this book is about individual women and their individual experiences of childbirth and poverty at the end of the twentieth century. In the chapters that follow, their stories will unfold. The stories are framed in the context and in the relevant literature; the stories, observations and insights are not in isolation but are part of a context: the social, political and economic context of their lives. In chapter one, I set the scene and explain why I felt that it was important to study childbearing women and poverty. I describe the local scene for the study and consider how the welfare state has defined women and how these definitions of women have shaped policymaking. I discuss the Beveridge Plan and its attack on want and poverty. I consider the demands of the feminist movements and their influence on the policy agenda. I consider the complexities of defining and measuring poverty and the incidence and extent of poverty in Britain. I briefly consider the tensions inherent in New Labour's Third Way proposals and the confusion and contradictions that surround women as dependents, carers and the 'undeserving' recipients of benefits.

In chapter two I explore the concept of poverty, its definition and meanings.

I explore the incidence and extent of poverty in the UK and explore some theories and explanations for the causes of poverty.

The process of the research is described in chapter three. I describe the methodology, explore the definitions of ethnography and discuss the process of analysis and some of the issues of doing fieldwork. I debate the use of interviews as a data-collection tool and consider the tensions around issues of truth, objectivity and trustworthiness in ethnographic research. As part of the ethnographic study method, it was necessary to be part of the community where the study took place. The research was carried out by a white, female, middle-class (as defined by occupation) researcher, who is also a practising midwife and employed in an academic post. As such, the life style, living standards, freedom and experiences of the researcher are far removed from the lives of the women in this study. Throughout the study, the aim has been to be reflexive, acknowledging the fact that the researcher is part of the world being studied. It reflects and is shaped by the conscious beliefs, values and experience of the researcher. As part of the reflexive process of feminist research, these beliefs, values and experiences must be explored; anger about injustice and inequality, together with childhood experiences of poverty, are part of the researcher and thus are part of this work. Throughout the research, the aim has been to see the world from the perspective of those women living and experiencing childbirth whilst living in poverty. The style has sought to recognise that differences between the researcher and the researched do exist, but by establishing a relationship with the women, it became possible to document women's own accounts of their lives and experiences. Ann Oakley explains in 'Interviewing Women':

'The goal of finding out about people through interviewing is best achieved when the relationship of the interviewer and interviewee is non-hierarchical and when the interviewer is prepared to invest his or her own personal identity in the relationship' (1995:41).

The interviewer nearly always has more power than the interviewee: the interviewer asks questions, probes and investigates; the women in the study responded willingly and openly. Many of the women I interviewed in the course of this research became friends. They welcomed me into their homes, they offered me food and beverages, and they gave me their time and were willing to share intimate and private details of their lives. In return, I listened, gave advice if asked and, according to some women, gave them the opportunity to talk to another adult. The lives of these childbearing women living in poverty were often stressful and, in many respects, lonely. These women shared aspects of their lives with their own mothers but there was evidence that female poverty and pregnancy increased social exclusion. These women did not join societies or clubs, they did not go to the theatre or the cinema, they did not go on holiday or have day trips away. Their lives revolved around their home, their children and, in most cases, their own mother.

Chapter four is called 'Exploring Motherhood: Responsibility and Respectability in Middleton'. It explores the recurring themes of responsibility and respectability and the meaning of motherhood for this group of women. I consider how middle-class discourses are used to construct the social codes for other classes and use interview data to explore some women's feelings about motherhood. I explain how some women in the study balanced the needs of their children with the demands of a life dominated by poverty and how being a 'good mother' brought satisfaction, respectability and a sense of personal worth.

In chapter five, I examine how individual women with different experiences and backgrounds find different ways of managing their lives as mothers, daughters, and as childbearing women living on state benefits. The chapter is called, 'Becoming Respectable and Sharing Responsibilities: Grandmothers, Networks of Support and the Search for Social Inclusion'. I examine the importance of Christmas and the significance of exotic pets as well as the realities of managing food and shopping on an inadequate income. National statistics alone cannot tell the full story of poverty. It was not difficult to see how in small areas individuals suffer many disadvantages simultaneously. The women in this study had no paid work, no bank accounts, no access to credit, no household, buildings or contents insurance; they lived in poor housing without central heating, over half experienced ill health in the previous year, and they took no part in the social or political life of the community. Drugs and crime were major areas of concern but, in particular, the crime of domestic violence had a major impact on the lives of many of the women who contributed to the study. Using field notes, observations and other sources the stresses and strains of living in poverty are explored. Rather than describing a homogeneous culture, I attempt to see aspects of life from the perspective of the individual.

In chapter six, I explore the changing and varied nature of the relationships between childbearing women living in poverty and the men in their lives. Many of the women living in poverty, who shared their thoughts and feelings with me, were living in 'on and off' relationships with men. Sometimes they were married, sometimes cohabiting, sometimes single, often alone and unsupported by men. Their lives were very different and their relationships complex; the women had found very different ways of resolving the challenging issues in their relationships. They balanced the need to conform and be respectable with the need to regain control over their lives. They found individual solutions to their individual and disparate lives.

This book, like life, is filled with contradictions. A phrase that I often heard, and I return to this in later chapters, was *'no wage, no use'*; for women, the value of a man was measured in terms of his economic power. Some women saw the solution to the financial hardships of their life being in having a man who would provide for them. This was not often a feasible option. Yet another contradictory message that I often heard was *'any man is better than no man'*. The drive to conform, to be seen as 'respectable', meant that to be living in partnership with a man was always better than not, even if that man was abusive, unemployed or unfaithful.

I have called chapter seven, 'Domestic Abuse: Different Women, Different Problems and Different Solutions'. It examines domestic violence and considers how different women deal and respond to this issue during their childbirth experience. Domestic violence was a key, recurring theme; there was overwhelming evidence that it was a significant issue in many women's lives. Yet I found that there was no universal experience of violence, no universal response and certainly no universal solution to a common issue. I focus on one woman's story to illustrate the unique nature of a violent relationship and the complexities that surround one woman's attempts to survive. Dawn's story demonstrates how one woman was able to put her children first and how she responded to the external pressure to be respectable. I explore the reasons why some women stay in abusive relationships and the tactics that some women use to cope with violence.

In chapter eight, I consider the issues that surround 'Pregnancy, Poverty and the Health Professional'. It was evident in the study that some women felt that the care they received from midwives, doctors and others was dictated by their status and social class. I explore the concept of social class and challenge the assumptions that individuals in a social grouping are all the same. I consider the use of social class in defining and measuring health inequalities and the impact that such inequalities might have on both midwives and the childbearing women. I explore the attitudes of some midwives towards women in this study and consider how midwives perpetuate structures and stereotypes as a means of control and to exert their superiority and power.

The final chapter, chapter nine, draws together the key themes, issues in the research, and offers some advice to midwives about improving care. I also make some suggestions for further areas for research. In the conclusion to this study, it seems obvious that midwives, as key health-care professionals, should adopt feminist poststructural beliefs and try to learn to treat women as individuals with individual experiences and requiring individual responses to their needs.

This book, then, is a search for meaning: by listening to women, I sought to understand what childbearing and poverty might mean to individual women in this group. Just as there is no universal experience of childbearing and poverty, there is no universal solution. I have tried to avoid the temptation to look for quick-fix answers but I recognise that the women in this study shared some common issues. I felt that they all had insufficient material resources, and the lack of resources meant that they had no part to play in the normal activities associated with membership of society, but they were also all women – which, as will be seen, in some ways compounded their disadvantage. As women and as mothers I felt that they were socially excluded and unable to exercise all the rights associated with citizenship. I believe that all the women in this study needed more money to survive, to feed their children and to find a way into an inclusive society. They also needed to be treated as individuals and with respect.

In the first chapter I will begin by explaining why I chose to study childbearing women and poverty.

Poverty: a woman's issue

Why study childbearing women and
  poverty?
The local framework: poverty in the
  West Midlands, Great Britain
Women, poverty and ill health
Defining women: the role of the
  welfare state

Beveridge to the Third Way
Influencing the policy agenda
Women and the challenge of poverty
Not just a UK issue: the global
  framework
Responsibility, respectability and
  women's lives

In this chapter, I begin by explaining what led me to research childbearing women living in poverty. I then begin to describe the settings of the study. I describe the local framework and explain why I chose Middleton. I begin the focus on women; I argue that it is women who bear the brunt of poverty and who manage poverty on a daily basis. I was faced with undeniable statistical evidence and research reports that convinced me that there were compelling reasons to study childbearing women and poverty. I explore how the welfare state has defined women and how these definitions have shaped policymaking. I will discuss the Beveridge Plan and its attack on the 'five giants' of want, disease, ignorance, squalor and idleness and trace the history of the development of social policy from the Beveridge Plan to the Third Way. I will explain how poverty is a far more significant issue for women, especially childbearing women, than for the men in their lives. I will consider how female poverty is lost in general debates about women and consider the dangers of assuming that poverty is the same for all men and women. Having explored poverty historically, nationally and internationally and also in policy terms I then return to the women of Middleton. I conclude the chapter by beginning the exploration of poverty and respectability in women's lives.

WHY STUDY CHILDBEARING WOMEN AND POVERTY?

I chose to study childbearing women because I am a midwife and have a professional interest in the needs and care of women during their pregnancies and childbearing experiences. In the Introduction I explained how I felt that childbearing women living in poverty were a neglected group. I was motivated to undertake this research because I believed childbearing women who lived in poverty had been neglected and even shunned by the midwifery profession. I felt that the medical, nursing and midwifery literature that was readily available to midwives and students tended only to reflect the needs and experiences of white, middle-class, articulate women. These views are purported to be the voices of all childbearing women.

In chapter one I will set out some of the issues and events in my life that have influenced my thinking and have helped to form my beliefs and values. Like the women who have contributed to this study I am an individual, shaped by many events and influences. I am a white, middle-class woman; my experiences are not representative of all women but they have shaped my understanding. I share being a woman with half the human race, but like Spelman (1988) I reject the phrase 'as a woman' as the Trojan horse of feminist ethnocentrism. To focus on women 'as women' has traditionally addressed only one group of women: the white, middle-class women of western industrialised societies. Just as not all women are oppressed by sexism, not all women are abused, and not all women are happy to be mothers; their experiences and mine are all different. I present this research not 'as a woman', but as an individual who is interested in how women are alike and how they are different. I am interested in how women see and cope with their experiences and I am interested in their similarities and their differences. I bring these experiences, values and beliefs to the research process. It is these experiences and beliefs which have influenced my 'way of seeing' and shaped my interpretation, my intuition and understanding of the world. These influences have shaped the ethnography that follows.

Like Jean Orr (1997:74), I became a feminist before I knew the word. As a child, whilst my brothers were given every opportunity to further their education, I was told to study cookery as a certain way of catching and holding on to a man. When I trained as a nurse, and later as a midwife, I became increasingly aware of women's oppression. I saw women as the victims of domestic abuse as they sought treatment in accident and emergency departments. I saw them blame themselves for the attacks made upon them. In childbirth, I witnessed them being mistreated by some medical men, and saw a total lack of respect for their bodies, and their views and opinions unheard or dismissed as irrelevant. I trained as a student in the medicalisation of birth and watched as women were duped into believing that induction, augmentation of labour and operative deliveries were in their best interest. I watched women's experiences being devalued and their dignity in labour ignored. I saw the actions of midwives as they colluded with the establishment to treat women in childbirth as components on a production line (Hunt and Symonds 1995).

When, in the early 1980s, as an interested professional, I read Ann Oakley's work on housewives (1974), I knew that my education had only just begun, and that there was another way of understanding the position of women in society. Around the same time, I experienced the totally medicalised birth of my own two children and I read Oakley's work (1979) on becoming a mother. In 1981, I briefly joined the Greenham Common Women's Peace Camp, and in 1982, I was one of the 30,000 women to encircle Greenham Common. At that stage, I knew I was angry about women's oppression, but feminist theories were not part of the everyday life of a staff midwife. It was difficult to articulate the anger, or to attempt to construct another explanation of the world in which I was living. I knew that the people most likely to succeed to the higher echelons in nursing were men. I knew I felt deeply uncomfortable about changing my name and losing my identity when I married. I could not tolerate financial dependence on any man, nor what I perceived as a lack of control over my own life; thus I returned to paid work as a midwife and later as a teacher. Although I did not understand it at the time, the three classic feminist positions defined in the 1980s – radical, socialist/Marxist and liberal feminisms – provided an explanation of my world, and I began to believe that education was the solution. It is almost inevitable, then, that those feminist theories provide the theoretical lens or the philosophical underpinning for this study.

I had been brought up in an ordinary, working-class family, which struggled to make ends meet, with five children and a low income. My father worked long hours as a shop manager, and my mother had a part-time job, selling vegetables in a local greengrocer. I played a major role in the upbringing of my sister, who was ten years younger than I, and was responsible for most of the cooking, all of the cleaning, and the washing for all members of the family; and this was whilst my three brothers went out to play. Like Virginia Woolf, I was not afforded the privilege of 'a room of my own' (1929/1994) but, without a television or other means of entertainment, I read everything I could from the local library. At 17, I left home and began nurse training.

These reflections are included to offer some explanation as to why I see the world as I do. It is an attempt to examine my motivations and explanations of the world I am studying. Writers like Patricia Collins (1991) have argued that to make legitimate knowledge claims, researchers should have lived or experienced their material in some fashion. I am a woman, a mother, a wife and I have had some experience of living in poverty. Stanley (1985) advises researchers to explore their 'intellectual autobiographies' and the role of their emotions and feelings in the research process. Whilst this can be considered a high-risk procedure, I considered it essential. Sasha Roseneil (1993) writing about her experiences at Greenham Common takes a similar risk. She has exposed many of her individual thoughts and feelings and, in my view, has produced a more reflective and sensitive ethnography in the process.

In those early days, I think I was best described as an angry radical feminist. However, it became clear that anger was not enough and that there was a need to move on in my thinking and my analysis. What I did not realise was that I had moved to a poststructuralist kind of feminism. I had always felt uncomfortable about generalisations about the condition and position of women; I had always felt that midwifery as a profession failed when it ceased to see women as individuals with individual needs and experience. My early writings in midwifery had a common theme that urged midwives to look beyond the external and outward signs and see women as unique and special. This latest research has enabled me to set my philosophy of midwifery in a robust theoretical framework; this has been its raison d'être and its contribution to midwifery knowledge.

THE LOCAL FRAMEWORK: POVERTY IN THE WEST MIDLANDS, GREAT BRITAIN

The data for this study were collected in the suburbs of Walsall; to preserve the anonymity of the respondents I have called the district 'Middleton'. The area was easy to reach and had some of the most helpful community midwives around. They willingly acted as advocates, taxi drivers and facilitators for the research. They worked closely with the local GP and health visitors and helped to make the research happen.

Walsall is a metropolitan borough in the West Midlands, part of the United Kingdom. It is located to the north west of the Birmingham conurbation, and historically forms one of the Black Country districts. Until the early 1980s, the coal mining industries were the main sources of employment in the region. Walsall has a multicultural urban population of 260,000 people, with the population density greater in the western half, which was the former centre of heavy industry and manufacturing. According to the Director of Public Health, Walsall has higher unemployment, more people from ethnic minorities, and greater levels of deprivation than the national average (Walsall Health Authority 1997/98). More than 23 per cent of the population are under 15 years of age, and 12 to 15 per cent are over 65 years of age. Within the West Midlands, Walsall is ranked as the fifth most deprived district and, according to the Jarman score, Walsall is the 46th most deprived health district in England. Low birth weight, a result of poor uterine growth or premature birth, is higher in Middleton than in other West Midlands regions. However, perinatal mortality rates, i.e. stillbirths and first-week deaths, are surprisingly lower than the national average. In 1997, the perinatal mortality rate for Middleton was 7.6 per thousand births. This compares well with the West Midlands rate of 9.7 and the rate for England and Wales, which was 8.4 per thousand births. Infant mortality has also decreased in this area, and is below the regional and national rates.

According to the *Annual Employment Survey* in 1998 (Walsall MBC 1998), 38 per cent of the jobs in Walsall were in manufacturing. This compares with only 18 per cent in Great Britain. A quarter of all working women worked in manufacturing, and one fifth of the work force were women working part time. In 1996, the unemployment rate in Middleton was more than 26 per cent, which along with St Matthew's makes it the ward with the highest unemployment rate in the borough. In February 1998, at the time of this study, five and a quarter million people in Great Britain were receiving income support or income-based Job Seekers Allowance (*Social Trends* 28, ONS 1998b). In Walsall, 28,886 people were in receipt of such benefits; this represents 18.8 per cent of the population, as compared with 15.7 per cent of the population of Great Britain (Walsall Council Benefit Service/Benefits Agency Report 1998). These figures could be even higher, as the government estimates of take-up of income support are that between 20 and 26 per cent of those entitled to benefit are not claiming it; this suggests that 10,000 to 13,000 Walsall residents and their dependants are missing out on benefits (Department of Social Security [DSS] 1998). In 1997, the Walsall Anti-Poverty Unit demonstrated the extent of under-claiming by increasing the benefit receipt in the borough by £3/4 million, in the 11 months to November 1997. In the groups receiving income support, 17 per cent of the recipients were lone parents. The Walsall Council Benefit Service has indicated that 19 per cent of households in the borough were dependent on income support, and there has been a 31 per cent increase in the number of owner-occupiers receiving income support in the past four years.

The *Labour Force Survey* (ONS 1998a) has not produced unemployment figures for Walsall since 1996-97. It is argued that the numbers gathered for the surveys locally are not high enough to make reliable estimates. The 'claimant count' method relies on the numbers registering unemployed and claiming Job Seekers Allowance. According to the West Midlands Low Pay Unit, this method of counting substantially underestimates the true level of unemployment amongst women. Women who want to work may not claim Job Seekers Allowance if their partners are working, if they have caring responsibilities, or if school hours and school holidays restrict them. The strict 'actively seeking work' rules also discourage women from applying for state benefits; as such they are lost from the system of recording the numbers of claimants. In July 1998, the 'claimant count' of unemployment in Walsall was 6.6 per cent of all those in the labour market. This is over a third higher than for Great Britain. In January 1998, the level of those registered unemployed and claiming Job Seekers Allowance was 7.4 per cent in Walsall, and 5.2 per cent in Great Britain. In some wards, for example St Matthews, the figure was 18.5 per cent, more than three times the national average, and in Middleton, where this study was carried out, the figures were double the national average at 10.4 per cent. The claimant count was 15.1 per cent.

Wages in the West Midlands are at 95 per cent of Great Britain levels. However, women's wages are lower, at 92.8 per cent of the rate for Great Britain. Wage inequality for women is greater in the West Midlands than it is nationally. National average full weekly time earnings in 1996 were

£351.70. In Walsall, it was £300.90, i.e. 86 per cent of the national average. Walsall had the lowest gross full-time wages in the seven West Midlands County local authority areas; the lowest paid are worse off in Walsall.

In 1998, Walsall Metropolitan Borough Council undertook a 'Needs Appraisal' as part of its Housing Investment Programme. It stated that there was a considerable problem of disrepair and poor housing conditions in both private and public sector housing. Nine out of ten local authority dwellings were said to be in need of renovation. In the private sector, 12,500 dwellings were unfit. The housing stock is outdated, with 40 per cent built before 1950. The Townsend Score reflects material wealth, and is commonly used to measure deprivation. It is particularly appropriate for reflecting differentials in urban populations. It is derived from four area variables in the last 1991 census. These are:

1. Percentage of economically active residents, aged 16 to 59-64, who are unemployed.
2. Percentage of private households without a car.
3. Percentage of private households that are not owner-occupied.
4. Percentage of private households with more than one person per room.

Areas with negative scores have less deprivation than average; those with a positive score have more deprivation than average. Middleton had a score of 7-9. This was the highest score in Walsall.

In 1996, Walsall Health Authority, with the West Midlands Regional Health Authority, conducted a life-style survey in Walsall. This survey, *The West Midlands Life Style Survey 1996*, considered many aspects of life style and behaviour. Of particular significance was a prevalence of smoking study. In Walsall, the prevalence was 27.9 per cent, as compared with 26 per cent in the West Midlands. The highest percentage of smokers was found in Middleton, at 37.5 per cent (in this research over half of the sample of women were smokers). In the same survey, it was found that 20.2 per cent of the people of Walsall did not eat fresh fruit at least once or twice per week. In Middleton, more than 25 per cent of those responding ate fresh fruit less than once or twice per week.

Information from the 1991 census was used to measure the incidence of limiting long-term illness (LLTI). Walsall had a slightly higher rate than the West Midlands as a whole; 13.3 per cent as compared with 12.1 per cent. Middleton had the highest proportion of people with LLTI, at 17.1 per cent. The same survey asked people to describe their health; 29.4 per cent of the people of Walsall described their health as 'fair', 'bad' or 'very bad'. The average West Midlands response was 26.5 per cent. In Middleton, the figure was 37.7 per cent, exceeded only by Bloxwich East. The figures for deaths from coronary heart disease (CHD) reflect the deprivation scores. CHD is the major cause of death in Walsall; it accounts for one third of all male and one quarter of all female deaths in the borough. There is no doubt about it; I was researching in one of the most deprived areas of the UK.

WOMEN, POVERTY AND ILL HEALTH

In the research reported here, two thirds of the women reported ill health in the previous year; this was before the adverse effects of their current pregnancy. They complained of a wide range of illnesses from urinary tract infection to cancer of the cervix (see 'Introducing the Women'). Bunting (1997) argues that the proportion of adults reporting ill health increases with decreasing socio-economic status. The exception is acute sickness, which shows no socio-economic pattern for men or women. GP consultations increase with decreasing socio-economic status. The use of preventative services such as dental attendance and the use of ophthalmic services also decreases with socio-economic status. The women in this study often complained of ill health. They frequently visited the GP, but never visited a dentist or optician. The evidence from this study confirms the so-called 'Inverse Care Law': the availability and uptake of health services is less in areas where they are most needed (Hart 1971).

MacArthur *et al.* (1991) first documented the occurrence of substantial physical postpartum morbidity. The study of over 11,000 women identified widespread morbidity starting after childbirth. As many as 47 per cent of women reported one or more of a list of 25 health problems beginning for the first time after birth and lasting for more than six weeks. In a subsequent study by Bick and MacArthur (1995) it was found that many women suffered symptoms daily, some of which had a significant effect on various aspects of their lives. It was concluded that childbirth makes some women ill, and it is more likely to make them ill if they are poor. Whilst it could be argued that there has been a general upturn in some women's fortunes with better educational opportunities, equal opportunities legislation and reduced discrimination in the work place, these are not universal benefits to all women. The women who contributed to this study were outside the labour market and thus excluded from the benefits of the upturn. Walby (1997) also argues that women who are pregnant, women with small children, women from minority ethnic groups and those who have missed out on education have been marginalised and excluded. Lone parents without employment are still likely to be very poor. Women from minority ethnic communities are still likely to be unemployed. The ONS (1998b) states that in 1996, lone parents headed 21 per cent of all families, but in 90 per cent of cases, the mother headed lone-parent families. It appears that often female poverty is hidden, underestimated and makes women sick. It is women who bear the brunt of poverty, it is women who manage poverty on a daily basis and it is women who struggle to feed, clothe and house themselves and their children. In a predominantly patriarchal society, it is women who are excluded from full citizenship by their economic dependence on men and, according to Ruth Lister (1997), it is women who will continue to be disadvantaged by the polarisation of the labour market as they take up unskilled and low-paid jobs. All these statistics, reports and views seem to point in the same general direction; they reveal fundamental facts about some women in poverty. For me these are compelling reasons to study childbearing women and poverty.

DEFINING WOMEN: THE ROLE OF THE WELFARE STATE

Central to this book are women: women struggling to survive, make ends meet and make sense of their lives and experiences. First it is necessary to look more closely at women and in particular how they are defined by welfare and state policymakers. The position of the women I worked with was shaped by many influences: the state, society, the welfare and benefit system, traditions and cultures. They did not exist in a vacuum but were part of a society. The women in this study were at the forefront of poverty in the late twentieth century. Charles (2000) argues that it is not poverty itself that deprives women of citizenship but the gendering of citizenship rights. Accesses to social rights of citizenship are based on male patterns of employment in the public sphere. It is assumed that women's and men's rights are different because their patterns of employment are different. The social policy agenda is crucial in defining citizenship and in order to set the scene and contextualise the empirical data of the later chapters, a feminist analysis of contemporary policy debates is essential.

So now some history; how did we get to this place? It has been argued that to understand the present we have to have some idea of the past. It is necessary then to consider briefly the birth of the welfare state and the beliefs about women that were held at that time and subsequently. The Beveridge Plan was important in that it recognised that women had rights, linked firmly with responsibilities, and these philosophies formed the foundations of social policy and are still exerting their influence today. Women occupy a contradictory role in social policy and the debate continues to centre on the ways in which women should be defined.

BEVERIDGE TO THE THIRD WAY

In June 1941, Sir William Beveridge was asked by Arthur Greenwood, the Labour Minister for Reconstruction, to chair an interdepartmental committee on the co-ordination of social insurance. His initial analysis found that seven different government departments were directly or indirectly involved in providing cash benefits of one kind or another. War victims were helped by the Ministry of Pensions, but civilian disabled, widows and orphans were the responsibility of the Minister of Health. The Home Office was involved in workmen's compensation, and health insurance provided a panel of doctors for those in work. Wives and children were excluded. Sickness benefit was provided by 'approved societies', and local authority committees, the inheritors of the Elizabethan Poor Laws, paid means-tested benefits to those in need. His report set out why the nation needed a national health service, tax-funded allowances for children and full employment to make social security work. The 200,000-word *Social Insurance and Allied Services* (Beveridge 1942) was published in December 1942 with a 20-page introduction and summary available at 3d (old pence). Beveridge used three guiding principles. First, that 'a revolutionary moment in the world's history is a time for revolutions not patching'. Second, his plan for security of income, social security, was principally an attack on want. *Want*, he said, was only one of the five giants on the road to reconstruction and in some ways the easiest to attack. The others were *disease, ignorance, squalor* and *idleness*. Third, he stressed that social security must be achieved by co-operation between state and the individual. To make it all work Beveridge wanted family allowances, a national health service and 'maintenance of employment'. Timmins (1996) argues that in his attack on the five giant evils, Beveridge encapsulated much of post-war aspiration.

Thus, the Beveridge Plan (1942) laid the basis for the structure of health and welfare policies in post-war Britain. It was based on a very specific definition of a family as having a male breadwinner and a female unpaid carer within a married relationship with the financial responsibility for the wife and children being that of the man, and the care of the children and elderly or sick relatives being that of the woman. Women were clearly defined in relation to men with men as the sole provider for the family. The Beveridge Plan reflected the dominant ideas of the time on the 'naturalness' of gender roles and on the role of men as wage earners and women as mothers and carers who were financially dependent upon male wage earners (Symonds and Hunt 1996). These beliefs formed the structure of the welfare benefit system. The dual insurance system described how married women would be wholly dependent upon their husbands' national insurance contribution for any benefits. Marriage would be women's sole occupation. Timmins argues that in some ways, Beveridge's proposals improved the lot of women. Before his report, single women had virtually the same rights as men to unemployment benefits if in work, but only means-tested assistance if they had never worked nor paid any contributions. On marriage, women became 'adult dependents' on their husbands and, apart from maternity grants, they had no rights under the health insurance scheme.

Employment of women has always been an issue for the welfare state. In post-war Britain there was an expanding economy based on consumer capitalism and the expanding welfare state. The effect was an acute labour shortage that was met by women joining the work force along with workers from the commonwealth countries. In 1939 and 1943, women were rapidly joining the work force in both industry and the armed forces. Women, then as now, met with frustration and strain. Women being exhorted to participate in employment and at the same time being expected to care for their families and children is described by Charles (2000) as 'schizophrenic policy'.

In 1940, the qualifying age for women's pensions had been reduced to 60 to encourage them to undertake war work. Beveridge assumed along with many others that after the war women would return to their homes and become housewives. The 1931 census, ten years out of date, but the best evidence available, had shown that seven out of eight married women did not work so Beveridge assumed that during marriage most women would not be gainfully employed.

Another of Beveridge's concerns was the assumed problem of the falling birth rate. During the 1930s the birth rate had fallen but in fact in 1942 it was rising, the result of record numbers of marriages on the eve of war and the sharp rise in illegitimacy. Beveridge saw the future role of women quite clearly. 'In the next thirty years, housewives as mothers have vital work to do to in ensuring the adequate continuance of the British race. With its present rate of reproduction, the British race cannot continue' (1942:53, para 117). He not only expected married women to be housewives, but also wanted incentives for marriage and childbearing. He recommended a marriage grant, maternity grant and maternity benefit for 13 weeks for those in work, family allowances and widows' benefits. Women and children were to be able to use the new, free, National Health Service. The plan was described as 'putting a premium on marriage, instead of penalising it' (1942:52, para 117). The role of women in the new post-war world was clearly described; women were to be dependent on men and supported by men and the state. In return, their task was to ensure a supply of children, properly cared for, for the next generation.

The contradiction in the definition of women is further seen in the role of women as workers. Whilst women were defined as mothers and carers, the government was encouraging women to enter the work force to meet the shortages. Women, argues Charles (2000), were constructed by government policy and by themselves as temporary workers whose prime responsibilities were to their homes and families. Since the introduction of the welfare state, women have occupied a contradictory role; are they primarily mothers and carers or workers?

Winston Churchill, despite the distractions of winning the war, was committed to social insurance with initially the Poor Law as a safety net. He coined the phrase 'from cradle to grave' and created a national insurance for all classes for all purposes. In 1944, the government produced White Papers on social security, the National Health Service and on employment policy. The Ministry of National Insurance was set up and the 1944 Education Act followed. There was a housing White Paper in March 1945 and in June 1945, the last act of the coalition government, the Family Allowances Act became law. This provided five shillings a week for a second child and all subsequent children to every family and was the first universal benefit of the modern welfare state. Family allowance was initially paid to ensure 'subsistence' both in and out of work but partly to encourage 'the more successful' in society to have more children. Family allowance, paid directly to women, and seen as 'wages for motherhood', was part of the larger movement in the education of mothers and the eugenic emphasis on improving the quality of the population. According to Timmins (1996), Beveridge clothed his recommendations for women in pro-marital and pro-woman rhetoric. He saw the proposals as giving women 'new economic status' and 'a new life in relation to social insurance'. He even considered a separation benefit to be paid to married women when marriages broke up, unless the woman was the 'guilty party'. This was never implemented. He did not formally oppose married women working, although the special lower rate of national insurance, which was an optional payment with lower unemployment and disability payments, assumed that the husband would be providing a home to live in. Work by married women was seen as 'intermittent' and not crucial to the family's financial survival. Timmins (1996) argues that although Beveridge may have seen the woman as 'a partner, part of the team', he disliked the concept of wives as dependents, and argued that women deserved rights for their 'vital unpaid service'. The Women's Freedom League (Abbot and Bombas 1942) did not agree and argued that his proposals left women, as before, dependent and not as partners. In a work-based scheme, founded on employee contributions, women who did not work were dependent on their husband's contribution.

Timmins (1996) argues that Beveridge attempted to reconcile a new universalism that stretched from cradle to grave. The system was to provide incentives to work, to save and to take individual responsibility, whilst at the same time checking abuse. This, combined with a desire to end poverty, still forms part of the social policy debate today. The battle for the balance between ending poverty and leaving room for private initiatives continues to rage.

Through the years that followed, different governments with different political persuasions sought to combat the five giants described by Beveridge. In 1944, the Education Act, known as the Butler Act, was passed as part of the war against ignorance and its implementation left to the incoming Labour government. Education for both boys and girls to the age of 15 became a reality. Finally, Beveridge believed that a comprehensive health service would underpin his social security recommendations. In 1944, the White Paper 'A National Health Service' was published. Aneurin Bevan was the Minister of Health in March 1946. He was responsible for publishing further documents on establishing a national health service. His proposals included the nationalisation of hospitals and a tripartite structure of services. The history of its development and Bevan's efforts to win over the medical profession are part of the history of the welfare state. The National Health Service Bill was drawn up in March 1946.

Beveridge did not use the word poverty throughout his plan; his use of the word 'want', it is argued, helped him win support for the plan (Timmins 1996). Thus, issues of measuring and defining poverty were avoided. Rent and housing costs were another of Beveridge's special problems; the proposal for a flat rate within unemployment benefit was dropped by the Labour government that followed.

Between 1948 and 1973, Britain enjoyed a sustained period of economic growth. Industries flourished and unemployment was comparatively low. In the 1950s housing was put at the top of the government's list of priorities, with hospitals, health centres, schools and books some way behind. Housing estates like Middleton were built by local authorities to provide housing for the workers in the local industries. The houses with gardens, indoor toilets and bathrooms were built in streets proudly named after English heroes. The leather factories and lock factories stood alongside the steel and coal industries providing near full employment for the population.

INFLUENCING THE POLICY AGENDA

Feminist social movements are said to occur in waves. Feminists have, according to Charles (2000), both engaged with the state and expected a response from it in relation to changing policies. In Britain, the first wave is dated from 1870 to 1930 and was concerned with women's political and property rights. The second wave emerged in Western Europe and North America at the end of the 1960s. During the 1970s, the feminist movement formulated their demands. These were for:

'Equal pay; equal education and job opportunities; free contraception and abortion on demand; free 24 hour nurseries; financial and legal independence; an end to all discrimination against lesbians and a woman's right to define her own sexuality. Freedom from intimidation by threat or use of violence or sexual coercion, regardless of marital status and an end to all laws, assumptions and institutions which perpetuate male dominance and men's aggression towards women' (Charles 2000:1).

These demands focused on the state, attacking its control of women's fertility, its construction of women as dependents of men and its control of female sexuality and implicit support for male violence against women. These issues are central to the research presented here. The effects of poverty on women, their role in relation to the men in their lives, their experience of the crime of domestic violence and their role as women and as mothers are each considered in the research.

WOMEN AND THE CHALLENGE OF POVERTY

From Beveridge to the present, all governments have concerned themselves, to a greater or lesser extent, with the 'problem' of poverty; this is not necessarily women's poverty but poverty generally. Feminist researchers such as Glendinning and Millar (1992) argue for policies that reduce women's dependence on men and increase their independent access to resources. They urge a move away from the concept of the male breadwinner and recognition in policy that men and women are breadwinners of equal status. Mayo and Weir (1993) on the other hand argue for better opportunities for training and better employment prospects. Increasing the wages to the low paid, a transformation of the gender divisions of labour within households, and free child care to enable women equal access to the labour market have all been suggested as possible solutions to the problem of women's poverty.

In this section, I have sought to explain how poverty is a far more significant issue for women, especially childbearing women, than for the men in their lives. Using feminist research on poverty I will demonstrate how the world's resources are unevenly distributed between men and women and that as a result poverty is much more likely to be experienced by women, and their children, than it is by men. Women's financial dependence on men renders them vulnerable to poverty as does the fact that women, alongside those from ethnic minorities and the disabled, are overwhelmingly concentrated in the low-paid sectors of the work force. According to Payne (1991), although the study of poverty has continued for more than a century, it has been gender-blind in that definitions and measurements have tended to focus on families or households, rather than on women. As a result, the impact on individual women is largely lost, as dominant definitions have had the effect of obscuring women's poverty and deprivation generally. In other words, in poor households, the extent to which women might experience greater poverty than other members of the family is completely lost. In the past, it has been assumed that poverty was equally shared by all household members, but there is evidence in this and other studies that women cushion men from the full effects of poverty. Women in this study appeared to experience poverty differently to the men in their lives. They were, as they explained, 'at the sharp end', managing poverty on a daily basis.

Much of the research also ignores the fact that poor households headed by women, in particular single-parent households, are significantly over-represented in figures of household poverty. Despite the gender-blind nature of many accounts of poverty, its definition, measurement, incidence, causes and explanations are clearly women's issues. There are considerably more women in poverty than men (DSS 1994, 1998) and access to the labour market is severely limited by dependent children. According to Oppenheim and Harker's calculations 59 per cent of adults supported by income support are women (1996:92) and in 1992 in the UK, 5.4 million women and 4.2 million men were living in poverty as defined as on or below the income support level. There is an assumption that feminisation of poverty is a fairly recent event. In fact, Corcoran *et al.* argued in 1986 that women and children have a much lower and unstable per capita family income over time and a higher risk of falling into poverty than do men. In 1992, Lewis and Piachaud wrote, 'the simple fact is that throughout the last century women have always been much poorer than men'. At the start of the century 61 per cent of adults on all forms of poor relief were women (1992:27). What has changed are the causes of female poverty and its visibility. In the early years of the century, married women whose partners were low paid and who had large families predominated amongst women living in poverty. This group was closely followed by widows and older women. Now female poverty is concentrated amongst lone women, especially the elderly. Women's poverty is increasingly visible partly due to the demographic changes, the increase in divorce and the increase in single-parent families headed by lone mothers. The women in this study had a choice of poverty through dependence on a man earning a low wage, poverty through dependence on state benefits, or poverty because of their low wages. Their responsibilities as mothers of young children excluded them from the labour market.

Lone parents, mainly because of their responsibilities in caring for children and the high cost of child care, are more likely to be poor. Other minority groups such as black and disabled women are also vulnerable (Amott 1990, Cook and Watt 1992, Lonsdale 1990, Roberts 1995). Likewise, women in the United Kingdom are more likely to suffer poverty than men, and throughout their lives are more vulnerable to poverty and deprivation (Payne 1991). According to the ONS (1998b), in 1996, 21 per cent of all families were headed by a lone parent – in 90 per cent of cases by the mother. The benefits system in Britain was designed on the assumption that married women would generally be supported by men, and by men who would be in full-time employment most of their working lives.

The underlying causes of women's poverty are that women are determined as the economic dependants of men both in the structure of the labour market and in the payment of wages and state benefits. Women become vulnerable to poverty when they become economically dependent on men and thus lose direct access to earnings in the labour market. Payne (1991) argues that women's vulnerability to poverty is the result of the myth that men are the providers and women often face the choice of poverty inside a relationship or outside. According to Walby (1997:64) women who are not participating in paid employment with the benefit of educational qualifications are likely to be poor and disadvantaged.

Lister (1997:173) reiterates the feminist argument that women were not treated as full and independent citizens with men in the Beveridge Plan. She argues that women's dependency is entrenched in social assistance schemes, which channel benefits through male 'heads of households'. According to Lister, the social citizenship rights of married and cohabiting women are mediated by their male partners, thus ceasing to be rights at all. In this way means-tested benefits fail to address or may even aggravate the problem of female hidden poverty. Even where benefits are paid to women, eligibility is based on a couple as a unit rather than the individual. Thus, the official statistics tend to underestimate the poverty gap, as the family or household as the unit of measurement does not take into account the hidden poverty that can result when income is not distributed fairly *within* a family. Lister (1997) argues that women's financial poverty also interacts with their time poverty, as they take on the main burden of debt and of mediating with welfare institutions. Women act as shock absorbers of poverty with consequential implications for their health.

Similarly, the United Nations (UN) *Human Development Report* (UNDP 1996) also notes that on the human development index, 'men generally fare better than women on almost every socio-economic indicator'. In seeking improvements, the report recognises that 'not much can be done without dramatic improvements in the status of women and the opening of economic opportunities to women' (1996). From a range of sources there is more and more evidence that women are disadvantaged simply because they are women.

Townsend (1979) and Graham (1987a) also indicate the crucial differences in the ways in which men and women view their earned income. Men often retain part of their earnings for personal consumption even when money is tight, whilst women tend to use their own earnings for household rather than personal expenditure (Brannen and Moss 1987, Pahl 1989). According to Glendinning and Millar (1992:60):

'Women bear the burden of managing poverty on a day-to-day basis. Whether they live alone or with a partner, on benefit or low earnings, it is debts which result when they don't. As more women and men lose their jobs, and as benefits are cut or decline in value, women are increasingly caught in a daily struggle to feed and clothe their families.'

These authors argue that it is not only the disparate levels of income which exist between men and women, but their access to income and other resources, the time spent generating income and resources, and the transfer of these resources to other members of the family that are significant. The CPAG (Child Poverty Action Group) Report (Oppenheim and Harker 1996) cites findings from a study by Webb (1993), which found that 71 per cent of the total numbers of people on low wages were women and two thirds of adults in the poorest households were women. He also found that women in these households had about half as much independent income as men, that is £99 per week compared with £199.50 per week. Women are more likely to be poor because of lone motherhood, marital and relationship breakdowns and old age. Payne (1991:47) argues that women who are poor are more easily counted and more readily observed, but the extent of the poverty women experience remains obscured by both poverty research and government statistics.

Ruth Lister (1997) in her book *Citizenship* has examined the themes of inclusion and exclusion, rights and participation. She argues that citizenship can be seen in terms of status, carrying a wide range of rights, involving general obligations, and political participation. She sees citizenship as a dynamic process and as a deeply gendered concept. Women, she argues, are excluded from full citizenship by their economic dependence on men. She believes that the increasing polarisation of the labour market, with its particular disadvantage of unskilled working-class women, is likely to be aggravated in the European Union under the impact of the Single European Market. She sees an intensification of the 'feminisation of poverty' and argues that central to women's claims for full citizenship are the issues of autonomy and economic independence. Poverty, argues Lister, is corrosive of citizenship both as a status and as a practice, undermining rights and the ability to fulfil the potential of citizenship.

Dahl (1987:91) describes the relationship between economic dependency and women's poverty. She argues that a 'minimum amount of money for oneself is a necessary prerequisite for personal freedom, self determination and self realisation'. She sees women's economic dependence on men as a moral problem both on an individual and societal level. She asserts 'access to one's own money should be considered a minimum welfare requirement in a monetary economy'. She believes that:

'An independent income of one's own is a prerequisite for participation in and enjoyment of life, privately as well as publicly. Lack of money, on the other hand, gives a person little freedom of movement and a feeling of powerlessness' (1987:111).

This sentiment becomes particularly relevant to the women in this study; when they lived alone they had an independent, if inadequate, income. That income gave them some power and some freedom.

Research by Cragg and Dawson (1984) and McLaughlin (1991) confirms the importance to many women of an independent source of income and has demonstrated how the unequal power relationship is experienced by many women as a lack of control over resources, a lack of rights and a sense of obligation and deference (Lister 1997:112). Lister also sees the distribution of resources within a family as a function of the power relationships that in turn reflect the relative economic resources each partner commands. Hirschman's framework (Hobson 1990) of 'exit' and 'voice' has been used to analyse this relationship. 'Exit' refers to the ability to opt out of an unsatisfactory situation and 'voice' refers to the ability to change it. When women have an independent income they have both a voice and an opportunity to exit. Hobson (1990:237) argues that the more dependent women are, the weaker their voice. The lower their earnings potential, the fewer the exit possibilities; and the fewer the exit possibilities, the weaker the voice. This framework is especially helpful in analysing women's response to domestic violence. Without an independent income, women had very little chance of exit or the ability to leave an abusive relationship. Trapped in an abusive relationship, it became clear that for some women, their voices were weakened. Although this theory is helpful, there is a danger that general concepts such as a lack of power, having 'no exit, no voice', are imposed on all women. In this study, I found different women, in different situations, finding different ways of dealing with a common issue. For the women who were abused physically and emotionally assaulted by men there was no simple theorising, no easy diagnosis, or treatment and solution. Their lives were complex, and there were many ways of understanding their situations and responses.

Despite my personal search for individual explanations and meanings, the published literature continues to make assertions about *all* women. For example, an important influence on the development of explanations of poverty is the recent changes in gender and employment. According to Walby (1997:1), fundamental transformations of gender relations in the contemporary western world are affecting the economy and all forms of social relationships. She sees both convergence and polarisation in the contemporary restructuring of gender relations. The convergence can be seen amongst young people where there is increased access to education and the labour market, but polarisation is occurring between women of different generations. The younger women gain qualifications and labour market positions that are out of reach to older women who have built their lives around a different set of patriarchal opportunity structures (1997:2). Walby (1997) demonstrates that whilst the structure of the typical household has changed, with increases in divorce and cohabitation, and the proportion of families headed by a lone parent has increased, women are more independent of men but poorer. The passing of equal opportunities legislation and subsequent policies adopted by employers has to some extent reduced discrimination in the work place, but there are continuing and new patterns of poverty and inequality, particularly for women who are outside the labour market. She argues that the massive changes that are taking place in women's employment and education are transforming gender relations but only for some women. She argues some younger women are taking up educational opportunities, using them to gain good jobs, and women are returning to work more rapidly after childbirth (1997:64). She points out that the upturn in women's fortunes is not universal; sidestepped are women who are pregnant, from minority ethnic groups and those who have missed out on education. Women in different ethnic communities have different priorities and opportunities that generate different sexual divisions of labour. She argues that the complex interventions of the state as a provider of minimal benefits interact in some households to discourage some women's employment. Lone parents without employment are still likely to be very poor and women from minority ethnic communities are more likely to be unemployed. Walby states that changes in the economy as a whole cannot be understood outside of an understanding of the transformations in the structures of gender relations – the change from private gender regime or private patriarchy to a more public gender regime or public patriarchy. The changes in the form of gender regime, she argues, give rise to new forms of opportunity and inequality (1997:65). Whilst there is no doubt that there is 'truth' in these assertions and relevance in these views, it is the individual and subjective accounts of women living in poverty that concern this research.

NOT JUST A UK ISSUE: THE GLOBAL FRAMEWORK

According to Glendinning and Millar (1992), Millar (1989) and Pahl (1989), women in the United Kingdom are more likely to suffer poverty than men. This is not, however, a purely British problem. According to the UN, women represent 70 per cent of the world's poor. In the United States, a disproportionate number of women are poor (Zopf 1989), whilst in Sweden women form the majority of those dependent on state support, and are more likely than men to have a standard of living which is below subsistence level (Vogel *et al.* 1988). Throughout the western world and the so-called 'developing countries', women are over-represented amongst the statistics for the poor (Payne 1991). Globalisation is probably one of the most significant developments of recent years. The lives of childbearing women living in poverty in Walsall in the late 1990s must be seen in the context of dramatic changes in the world. Increased prosperity and economic growth should have led to fuller choices for all people, but in many countries this has not happened. World merchandise trade has tripled, and global trade services have increased 14-fold. The flow of capital has opened the world to a global financial market. Whilst developing countries have seized globalisation as an opportunity, others have not. The poorest countries, with 20 per cent of the world's people, have seen their share of world trade fall from 4 per cent to less than 1 per cent in the past 20 years (Parsons 1998).

The *Human Development Report* (UNDP 1996) explores the nature and strength of the links between economic growth and human development in the last decade. It notes that, since 1980, there has been a dramatic surge in economic growth in some 15 countries, bringing rapidly rising incomes to many of their 1.5 million people. Over much of this period, economic decline has affected 100 countries, simultaneously reducing the incomes of 1.6 billion people. The report argues that, although many governments are aware of the economic stagnation, the full extent is too often obscured by the success of fast-growing countries. It is argued that, whilst the world has become more polarised, the gulf between the rich and poor has widened. The poorest 20 per cent of the world's people saw their share of global income decline from 2.3 per cent to 1.4 per cent in the past 30 years; meanwhile, the share of the richest 20 per cent rose from 70 per cent to 85 per cent. That increased the ratio of the shares of the richest and the poorest from 30:1 to 61:1. Increased polarisation is reflected in the growing contrasts in regional performance. Most of Asia experienced accelerating per capita income growth, but most OECD (Organisation for Economic Co-operation and Development) countries generally maintained slow but steady growth. Where the overall economy grows, it does not necessarily expand the opportunities for employment. In the OECD countries in 1993, the average unemployment rate was 8 per cent, ranging from 2.5 per cent in Japan, to 10 per cent in the United Kingdom. The report argues that fairer opportunities for women and better access to education, child care, credit and employment contribute to human development. 'Investing in women's capabilities and empowering them to exercise their choices is the surest way to contribute to economic growth and overall development' (UNDP 1996). Education, reproductive health and child survival all help lower fertility rates, and thus create the conditions for slower population growth and lower education and health costs in the long term. Globalisation has increased affluence but this affluence has benefited men the most.

RESPONSIBILITY, RESPECTABILITY AND WOMEN'S LIVES

Despite the politicians' demands for 'rights linked with responsibilities' the women in this study (and their mothers) had very clearly defined ideas as to their responsibilities. For politicians, the responsibilities of the population focus on paid work, not unpaid caring, and work is the route to rights and thus citizenship. Those claiming unemployment benefits, now called 'Job Seekers Allowance', are required to be available for work. The balance between rights and responsibilities is debated by Ruth Lister (1997). She argues that the overemphasis on paid work does not reflect the reality of gender relations. By not participating in paid work, the women in this study were not ignoring their responsibilities as citizens but were defining their own responsibilities to their children, home and families.

The women in this study clearly saw that they were responsible for their children's (and their grandchildren's) welfare and this is demonstrated throughout the research in a variety of ways. It was possible to see how, against all sorts of difficulties, these women put the needs of their children first. Their own needs always came second: they often wore second-hand clothes so that their children could have school uniform, they often went without food so that their children could eat, and often some women ate their children's leftovers rather than food of their own choice to save money. They saw responsibility as part of the parenting package; it was closely intertwined with love for their children, which was expressed in a variety of ways. For this group of women, poverty was constant but the ways in which they coped with the daily grind of poverty varied from woman to woman.

Responsibility or obligations are closely linked to the concept of respectability. Respectability requires a well-developed sense of responsibility and a sense of moral worth and value. Skeggs (1997) links the concept of respectability with that of class. She argues that respectability has always been a marker and burden of class, signifying a standard to which to aspire. The notions of the deserving and the undeserving poor are linked to the classification of respectable and the non-respectable. Respectability contains judgements of class, race, gender and sexuality. In chapter three we will explore some women's own analysis of this division and the use of their terms the 'working poor' and the 'smelly poor'. The working poor, not necessarily those working for monetary gain but working to keep their homes and children neat and in good order, were respectable whilst those who were classified as 'smelly poor' had not achieved respectability. The working poor believed that the midwives would treat them more favourably if they were 'clean', 'tidy' and respectable. They were very conscious of the midwives' attitudes towards them, especially when they visited the antenatal clinic or the hospital; they knew they were being 'weighed up' and the result of the assessment would determine the outcome of care. The search for respectability was part of the search for moral and personal worth.

Class, as a concept, has been almost totally removed from current social policy. In the 'Third Way' politics, class divisions are no longer discussed; the debates are around social exclusion, community integration and enabling policies. However, in a recent Mori poll (*Guardian* 22 August 2002) it is reported that more people are 'working class and proud of it'. Today 68 per cent of people see themselves as working class as opposed to 52 per cent in 1994. Certainly only 3.6 million of a work force of 28 million is now engaged in manufacturing. This *Guardian* leader writer argues that 'the plight of unskilled low wage families rightly worries New Labour ministers'. Cahill (1994) notes the widespread reluctance to use class in contemporary social policy. He says:

'Class is important in the distribution of life chances. Clearly social class matters in relation to education, health and housing and many people are aware of the differential advantages enjoyed by people from different class locations. But it is social class as an organising principle, as a unifying concept which is in sharp decline' (Cahill 1994:18).

However, Skeggs (1997) believes that class remains a central issue; it can shape and recreate women's experiences and social policy. According to Skeggs, respectability is central to the development of class categorisations. She says:

'Respectability is one of the most ubiquitous signifiers of class. It informs how we speak, who we speak to, how we classify others, what we study and how we know who we are (or not). Respectability is usually the concern of those who are not seen to have it' (1997:1).

Skeggs argues that it is because the working classes have been persistently classified as dangerous, polluting, threatening, pathological and without respect that respectability is an issue. The categories of deserving and undeserving poor as being homogeneous groups exert a powerful effect. The disreputable poor are seen as 'undeserving' of benefits, dishonest, feckless and lacking self-discipline, whilst the deserving poor (widows, orphans and those who cannot help their situation) are in another category and are somehow respectable. In this study many women were striving for respectability; they believed that if they achieved it they would receive better care and the approval of the health professionals. In chapter eight, it can be seen how midwives made assessments of and judgements about women using a range of criteria, but cleanliness, respectability and their rights to claim state benefits were important. Respectability, for the women in this study, meant belonging, inclusion, being accepted. They were uncomfortable when their life style was questioned, when their decisions to have children, live with their partners or live apart from their partners were challenged by health professionals. Being respectable meant they would be treated with respect, acknowledged and recognised as an individual. They were also acutely aware of how often they were not viewed as being respectable.

In the next chapter I will return to the issue of poverty, its explanations, definition, measurement and some of the solutions that are offered.

2

Making sense of poverty

Defining poverty
The measurement of poverty
The incidence and extent of poverty in
  Britain
Theories and explanations for the
  causes of poverty

The underclass debate
Communication, technology and
  information: new capital?
Current policy debates: the search for
  structural solutions
Social exclusion

In this chapter I begin by defining poverty and discuss how poverty is much more than physical needs and social standards; it is about rights, needs and political power. Income levels alone are inadequate in defining poverty. I then explore the ways in which poverty has been measured and consider the evidence of the incidence and extent of poverty in Britain. I then examine some of the theories and explorations of poverty and the debates around the terms class and underclass. I will then move on to discuss the policy debates and the search for structural solutions to poverty. I explore some of the tensions around the 'Third Way' proposals and the concept of social exclusion.

DEFINING POVERTY

It is important to define poverty but this is neither simple nor straightforward. The term is often avoided by politicians. The meaning of 'poverty' is controversial, as Roll (1992) explains: the word has a moral force and is used as a call to action. Poverty is about physical needs and social standards; it is about a shortage of money but also about rights, needs and political power. Roll explains that most experts agree that it is impossible to define poverty based on physical needs, observing the world or by asking the population its views. Measures of poverty do not tell the complete story: women, ethnic minorities, even the homeless are often excluded.

Donnison (1998) argues that 'poverty' is the word most often used by pressure groups in Britain to describe the trends they deplore. The groups make use of poverty statistics, which describe the growing numbers of individuals in poverty. Yet poverty itself is a complex concept; deprivation, hardship, exclusion, need, the poverty line, measures of inequality, and the Gini co-efficient (Hills 1996), which measures where a population sits on a scale from complete equality to complete inequality, are all used by academics and governments to grapple with the issue. Poverty pressure groups are naturally sympathetic towards those who are poor (e.g. Oppenheim and Harker 1996). Those who are unsympathetic (e.g. Green 1998) argue that poverty as such does not exist in Britain, only inequality, and the poor are only poor in relation to contemporary British standards. The stance taken in this study has been unequivocally one of sympathy and admiration for the women who, in making sense of a life lived in poverty, have provided the rich data and the opportunity to share in their lives. These of course are my values, the beliefs that have guided the study and shaped the research process.

Oppenheim and Harker (1996), writing for the Child Poverty Action Group, opt for two relatively simple definitions of poverty:

1. The numbers living on or below income support/supplementary benefit.
2. The numbers living below 50 per cent of average income after housing costs.

Definitions of this nature are factual and exclude any consideration of the effects of poverty on individuals and their families. Oppenheim and Harker (1996) offer a further and more thoughtful definition:

'Poverty means going short materially, socially and emotionally. It means spending less on food, on heating, and on clothing than someone on an average income. Above all, poverty takes away the tools to build the blocks for the future – your life chances. It steals away the opportunity to have a life unmarked by sickness, a decent education, a secure home and a long retirement' (1996:4).

These are some of the reasons why it is important to study the impact of poverty on individual lives and in particular the impact of poverty on women. The women in this study went without materially, socially and emotionally. They managed on a very tight budget, they 'robbed Peter to pay Paul', and managed to feed their children all of the time and themselves most of the time. They were frequently 'not too well'; many had a bad back or were depressed. They all wanted a decent home, enough money and perhaps the opportunity for their children to get qualifications and a good job.

Many texts begin with a simple description of *relative* and *absolute* poverty (e.g. Alcock 1997), but there is clearly a need to focus on a range of definitions that describes more than levels of income; aspects such as the features of life, life styles, possessions and social activities are also important. Some texts offer definitions of *subsistence* poverty, where individuals are unable to provide themselves with the basic needs of food, clothing and shelter, and *relative* poverty, which is defined in relation to the living standards of the population or particular group under discussion. Ackers and Abbott (1996), along with other authors, differentiate between *absolute* poverty, where individuals are unable to meet their basic needs of food, shelter and clothing (this usually describes those who are homeless and starving), and *subsistence* poverty, where individuals are unable to provide for themselves and their families with agreed basic requirements without assistance from the state or charities. *Relative* poverty is a more useful concept as it moves away from mere survival to considering such aspects as the quality of life. However, the term 'relative' is used in the literature in different and often conflicting ways. It can mean relative in historical terms, relative to other countries, relative to other groups, or relative to the prevailing living standards of other groups within a country. Townsend, in his major work on poverty in the UK, values the term 'relative', and states that poverty can be applied consistently and objectively only in terms of the concept of relative deprivation. He has most clearly described this notion of poverty in relation to a person's surrounding community and social networks:

'Individuals, families and groups in the population can be said to live in poverty when they lack the resources to obtain the types of diet, participate in the activities and have the living conditions and amenities which are customary or at least widely encouraged or approved in a society in which they belong' (1979:31).

Townsend (1979: 337) argues that 'to comprehend and explain poverty is to comprehend and explain riches'; thus as a concept, it is relevant only in relative terms. He clearly believes that poverty is more extensive than is generally or officially believed or recognised and is an inevitable feature of severe social inequality. He argues that it is the actions and desires of the rich to preserve and enhance their wealth so as to deny it to others; in addition any attempts to alleviate poverty must deal with the issue of the control of wealth and the control of institutions created by wealth (1979:891). His radical recipe for an effective assault on poverty is based on egalitarian assumptions and includes the abolition of excessive wealth, abolition of excessive income, the introduction of an equitable income structure and some breaking down of the distinction between earners and dependants.

On the other hand, Green (1998) argues that with any 'relative' definition of poverty some people will always be classified as poor; this statement justifies his belief that the extent of poverty has been exaggerated. Fundamental to this argument is that, short of absolute equality, it will be impossible to raise everyone above the poverty line, because the line moves up with prosperity and the poor will always be poor. Thus it is argued that the poverty line as such is an outdated and irrelevant concept.

In February 1999, the government, led by Tony Blair, announced that it would publish an annual audit on poverty. Howarth *et al.* (1998) describe 46 statistical indicators. These include income levels, economic circumstances, health, exclusion from work, education, social cohesion, crime and housing. Each indicator will serve as a base line for the present government's activity and will be used to measure progress and report on poverty and social exclusion. The latest report (Rahman *et al.* 2001) uses 50 indicators; this report is discussed later in this chapter.

Green (1998) argues that over recent years there has been a huge increase in the numbers of people who look to politicians and the state for the means of life. In 1950 about 4 per cent of the population relied on national assistance, whereas in 1998, 17 per cent of the population relied on income support. If other means-tested benefits are included, the figure rises to 27 per cent. These statistics support Green's argument; by producing a definition of poverty and developing policies based on that definition, this in turn inevitably leads to an over-dependent society.

George and Howards (1991) opt for a looser definition; they define poverty along a continuum of want that begins with starvation, moves on to subsistence, then to social coping and ends with social participation. They argue that in advanced affluent, industrial societies, poverty cannot be defined simply in terms of starvation or in terms of basic survival needs but that all definitions and measurements of poverty involve and incorporate, to a greater or lesser extent, the values of those defining the problem.

Deeply embedded in both the definitions and measurements of poverty is the assumption of the role of the man as the family breadwinner; indeed the benefit system was constructed on this assumption. The introduction of the Child Support Act in 1992 gave the Child Support Agency the power to trace the biological father and make him liable for the children regardless of the mother's wishes. Women were poor only when men failed to provide. Most writers on poverty, sympathetic or hostile, tend to assume that male and female poverty is the same thing, a view disputed by Ruth Lister (1997) and explored later in this chapter. Defining poverty is almost as complicated as measuring poverty; definitions and measurements are based on or avoided according to meanings that are ascribed to the condition. In the next section, I explore the ways in which poverty has been measured.

THE MEASUREMENT OF POVERTY

If defining poverty is difficult, it is equally difficult to measure. Even the Department of Work and Pensions has conceded that it is 'far from straightforward to measure poverty' (Walker 2002). Social researchers first began to measure the extent of poverty in the nineteenth century. The studies by Booth (1894) and Rowntree and Seebohm (1901) in the east end of London and in York were the first to attempt to set a poverty line by which differing grades of poverty could be calculated. Other studies at this time illustrated the cost of food, rent and necessities for a family on low income (Pember Reeves 1911). The measurement and definition of poverty have changed throughout this time, and are still subject to debate and change.

According to Piachaud (1987b), there are three approaches to the measurement of the poverty line. These are the professional or expert approach, the expenditure or consumption approach, and the public opinion or social consensus approach. The second method, the budget standard approach, was used by Rowntree in his study in York in 1899; he defined poverty in terms of a minimum weekly amount that was necessary to secure the necessities of life. Two further studies were carried out in 1936 and 1950 (Rowntree 1941, Rowntree and Lavers 1951) but so called non-essential items such as newspapers, books, radios, beer, tobacco, holidays and presents were included. The second approach was also adopted by Townsend (1979), who systematically measured how different groups of people live and spend their money. He defined income and expenditure much more widely than previously and in more wide-ranging groups of people and established a list of 60 indicators including amount of food, overcrowding, the ability to buy birthday presents etc. He concluded that there was a 'deprivation threshold' when participation in many of the 60 indicators dropped so sharply that the individuals concerned were not simply unequal but were in poverty (Townsend 1979:60).

Townsend's work has been subjected to much criticism. For example, Piachaud's (1981:32) criticisms focus on the use of indicators; he states 'it is not clear what they have to do with poverty, nor how they were selected'. He goes on to challenge the view that going without a Sunday joint and not eating fresh meat or cooked meals are necessarily associated with deprivation. He argues that choices of this nature may reflect differing cultural values. Wedderburn (1974) also criticises the index for its apparent arbitrary inclusion and exclusion criteria. These writers suggest that respondents found it impossible to distinguish between choosing not to purchase a particular good or service because they did not want or need it, and not purchasing it because it could not be afforded.

The concept of poverty, its definition and measurement are inevitably subjective. For the women in this study, some saw themselves as poor; others felt they were better off than others, so were not 'poor' as such, although they were indeed poor by standard definition. Definitions of poverty frequently result in blanket statements that ignore the effects of poverty on the individual and ignore the individual's own interpretation of their position and life style.

Townsend (1979:46) sought to define and measure poverty not 'as the unwitting servant of contemporary social values' but using a methodology which distinguished 'between objective and conventionally acknowledged poverty'. To some extent, Townsend can be seen to be caught in a dilemma; if he defined poverty according to public opinion then he was in danger of being dominated by the unacceptable values of the society. If he adopted a more academic approach he ran the risk of being in an 'ivory tower' and rejection on the grounds of being detached and irrelevant; either way he is still imposing structuralist generalisations upon a disparate group.

The social consensus or public opinion approach to defining poverty described by George and Howards (1991:16) measures poverty according to the views of the public. This method is subjective (although it purports to be objective) as the researchers, who are part of the public, inevitably frame the questions, probably guide the responses and thus to some extent define the results. This approach can lead to austere or generous definitions of poverty according to the state of public opinion. The approach is based on the belief that various items, goods and services should only be included in a poverty index if they are socially perceived to be essential. This will vary at different times. This public opinion approach argues that the public, presumably a representative sample, is the best judge of what poverty means (not an expert or a researcher). Such approaches are favoured because the results are more likely to influence governments when the public have power to elect or eject from office. A poststructural theorist would argue that all meanings are socially constructed, fluid and subject to constant reassessment and change. The researcher may not have the ability to stand outside and cannot assume objectivity.

A central criticism of the traditional measures of poverty is of the focus on the household as the unit of consumption. Poverty research has incorrectly assumed a division of resources within a household that is equitable and agreed a so-called consensus model of the family rather than a conflict model. Glendinning and Millar (1992) dispute such a model and suggest that the pattern of women going without or being denied equal shares existed and was well known at the beginning of the century. Women's experience of going without is seen as voluntary and even self-sacrificial, rather than imposed; as such, it is seen as a legitimate and even natural resolution to income difficulties. Government definitions of poverty also concentrate on income, presumed to be provided by the male head of household, rather than family expenditure and consumption as measures of poverty.

As can be seen, the problem with trying objectively to define poverty is that ideas of 'average' living standards are vague, and researchers, policymakers and others find it difficult to agree on what constitutes deprivation. In the 1980s, researchers working on a survey of *Breadline Britain* (revisited in 1990 and shown on London Weekend Television in 1992) gained a two-thirds consensus from a public opinion survey that a list of goods and services represented necessities for an acceptable standard of living. The list, described by Mack and Lansley (1985), included self-contained accommodation with indoor toilet and bath, weekly roast joint and three meals a day for children, money for public transport, heating and carpets, toys for children, money for Christmas, and a refrigerator and washing machine.

Mack and Lansley's (1985) study took account of many of the methodological criticisms of Townsend's work. They defined poverty in relative terms, but devised new ways of determining what were the necessities of life in modern Britain. They accepted Piachaud's (1981) criticisms that personal taste and cultural values might influence choice, and included a question relating to each respondent's view of what they lacked. They also excluded some items from the index that high-income groups were as likely, or nearly as likely, to say they lacked as poor-income groups – for example, the cost of a garden. Television sets were excluded because the numbers of individuals without this item were so few. Mack and

Lansley (1985) did not want to be accused of making arbitrary choices, assuming their methods were more objective, but they rejected Rowntree's use of experts and went further than Townsend's (1979) subjective choices. They claimed a large degree of consensus of public opinion as to the necessities of life, with a deprivation index consisting of 22 items. They defined poverty as an enforced lack of socially perceived necessities, calculated according to those who lacked three or more items from the index.

In 1983, the time of their study, and using this definition, there were 7.5 million people living in poverty, some 13.8 per cent of the population. By 1990, they found a substantial increase in poverty, again using their own definition; the numbers in poverty had increased from 7.5 million to 11 million. Those in severe poverty, defined as lacking seven or more items, had gone up from 2.5 million in 1983 to 3.5 million in 1990. However, the inclusion of new categories in the 1990 study makes comparisons of the two studies difficult.

Piachaud (1987b) criticises this study and argues that the list of necessities is still based on the researcher's judgements and other items could be included or excluded. Walker (1987) argues that Mack and Lansley's approach is unnecessarily simple and does not allow respondents to determine the *quality* of goods and services. Walker (1987) proposes that basic needs should not be determined by groups of experts but by panels of ordinary people who have had the opportunity for in-depth discussions. Thus, he favours the public opinion or consensus definition of poverty.

The definition of what constitutes poverty and how it should be measured remains a matter of debate. In the *Social Attitudes* survey (Taylor-Gooby 1990), only 25 per cent of the respondents were prepared to agree with the Townsend definition of relative poverty, with 50 per cent preferring the 'breadline' definition. However, there was a near unanimous agreement at 92 per cent on a definition of poverty as 'not having enough to eat without getting into debt', near the absolute or below subsistence definition.

In response to criticism of Townsend's work, which was said to blur the line between poverty and inequality, a model based more on social 'coping' has been suggested by George and Howards (1991). They argue that it is morally unacceptable for governments to define poverty in affluent societies in terms of starvation or subsistence. They suggest that the social coping definition, which sees poverty in relation to 'working class' standards and 'modest requirements', is more realistic and justifiable. They state:

'People in subsistence poverty for long periods may not necessarily be starving but their life is socially intolerable in advanced industrial societies for their standard of living is so markedly below that of the rest of society.

People are in poverty if their income and resources are not sufficient to provide them with those goods and services that will enable them to live a life that is tolerable according to working class life styles' (George and Howards 1991:6).

This 'social coping' definition is more generous and more open to dispute. Those undertaking the research and other outsiders will be bound to make value judgements as to what exactly are 'modest requirements'.

In 1991, Bradshaw and Millar defined and priced a basket of goods and services selected to represent a standard of living. The basket included the cost of video and television hire, essential food (at Sainsbury's prices), basic clothing (at C&A store prices), public transport and haircuts. However, goods such as alcohol, cigarettes, cosmetics, a freezer and an annual holiday were excluded. The study reported that more than 50 per cent of lone mothers and single pensioners failed to achieve the budget. The researchers' definition of a standard of living can always be criticised as being unrepresentative of the wants and needs of particular communities. Some of the women in this study expressed how good it would be to shop at Sainsbury's and buy clothes from C&A but this was not possible. Some explained that the usual place to buy clothing was the charity shops when cash was available and from shopping catalogues when it was not. Some women bought their children's clothing from the 'tat man', others from friends and family. Most women in this study purchased food on a daily basis from markets, and from shops such as Lidl, Kwik Save and other discount chains. In the published research the definitions of poverty influence the extent of measured poverty: the more 'charitable' the definition of poverty, the higher the rates that are reported. In this study, it is the impact of poverty on individuals that is considered important.

The European Economic Union defines the poor as those who have a disposable income of less than half the average equivalent disposable income per capita in their own country (Hantrais 1995). The definitions used in British government statistics have also been modified in recent years. Until 1988, the term 'low income families' was used, but this was abandoned in favour of the 'households below average income' scale (HBAI). By calculating households instead of families, the number of persons constituting a group became of great significance. The statistical effect was to reduce the numbers of people living 'below half the average income' by over a million. Green (1998), who is generally unsympathetic to arguments in support of the poor, believes that the HBAI scale should be discarded and replaced by a series of independent figures that highlight the success or failure of public policies in encouraging independence.

Government statistics as measures of poverty, such as the *Family Expenditure Survey*, are generally mistrusted and criticised (Miles and Irvine 1979). Oppenheim and Harker (1996) argue that, although the survey uses a large national sample (6,400 households per year), those living in the most severe poverty are likely to be excluded. For example, those living in bed and breakfast accommodation, hostels and institutions are excluded and this, together with the fact that those living in poverty are less likely to respond to official surveys, makes the information unreliable and the extent of poverty underestimated. Having considered the definitions of poverty and the attempts made to measure it, the incidence of poverty now has to be considered as part of the backdrop of this research.

THE INCIDENCE AND EXTENT OF POVERTY IN BRITAIN

Since the late 1970s, the gap between the rich and the poor in the United Kingdom has widened considerably, and according to Hills (1996:5) the growth of inequality in the UK has been faster than that of any other comparable industrial country. Despite variations in figures and definitions, the data suggest that the living standards of those in the bottom two or three tenths of the income distribution have failed to rise significantly, whilst those at the top of the distribution have risen much more rapidly than average. The nearer the top an income group lies, the faster its income has risen. Income distribution is analysed by the Department of Social Security (DSS), the Office of National Statistics (ONS) and the Institute of Fiscal Studies (IFS), all of which use McClements equivalence scales to take into account variations in the size and compositions of households. The DSS and IFS use both before and after housing costs scales, whilst the ONS only uses before housing costs scales. Information on the distribution of income is provided by the DSS using the households below average income (HBAI) definition. Two different measures are used: one before and one after housing costs are deducted. Housing costs consist of rent, water rates and community charges, mortgage interest, structural insurance and ground rent and service charges. Disposable income is defined as income after deductions of income tax and national insurance contributions. This of course applies only to earned income or declared income after the deduction of income tax and national insurance and ignores the black economy.

Average household disposable income is sometimes used as a measure of the standard of living. In 1996-97 non-retired households composed of three or more adults had an average disposable income of £560 per week. This compares with £415 per week for two-adult households and £270 per week for single-adult households. More significantly, in a family with two adults and two children the average disposable income in 1996-97 was £434. Thus the income in a household on half the average would have been £217 per week (*Social Trends* 28, ONS 1998b:93).

By 1995, it was reported that a third of households (27 per cent of all families) were in receipt of some form of means-tested benefits. In other words, they were deemed by official calculations to be entitled to benefits by virtue of the fact that their income was below the minimum level (*Social Trends* 28, ONS 1998b). In ONS 1998, it was reported that the proportion of people in the United Kingdom whose net household disposable income was below average rose from 59 per cent in 1979 to 63 per cent in 1994-95. The proportion of people below half of average income had doubled since the first half of the 1980s (ONS 1998b:100). Similar changes have occurred in the proportion of people with incomes below both 60 per cent and 40 per cent of average income. As can be seen, most attempts to measure poverty use household or family income or expenditure as the basis for calculating the extent of poverty. This incorrectly assumes that all individuals are equal recipients of income. Income and expenditure in households are public knowledge but what happens in families, and in particular to women, is considered a private matter. The extent and impact of poverty, as this study will demonstrate, is inextricably linked to the person who holds the purse strings. Poverty research has generally been 'gender-blind', assuming that poor women are just the wives of poor men. But poverty is clearly an issue that affects women in a major way.

In 1984 Hilary Graham was one of the first writers to expose the role of women in the family and describe the impact of poverty on mothers' abilities to care for their children. Her important work considered the role of women in organising their money, time and energy to promote the health of their families. She was able to demonstrate the unequal way in which resources are shared out amongst families with children and the impact of gender divisions and social class on health. At that time she stated that health policies based around responsibilities and choice must face the material realities in which parents work for better health; she argued that class structure and sexual divisions continued to shape the distribution of health resources and responsibilities. She concluded by saying that the fewest resources are allocated to those with the greatest responsibility.

In 1999, the position of women in Middleton was not dissimilar. Women, in their very different ways, faced the day-to-day reality of coping with poverty. Pahl (1989) also argued that women were more likely than men to spend any income they had on their children; women's wages, where they exist, are crucial for keeping families out of poverty. Women not only have less access to resources within households as compared with men but their responsibility for domestic labour and child care enhances men's earning power. According to Charles (2000) women's unpaid labour in the home helps to free their partners from caring and domestic activities, enabling them to engage in wage labour and increase their wages and/or career prospects. In this study, the men who were on low wages were free to work extra hours or do 'fiddles and foreigners' in order to increase their income. Men never had to pay someone to care for their children.

In 1988, the number of pregnant women on means-tested benefits was one in five; by 1994 it had risen to one in three (Maternity Alliance 1995). The Child Poverty Action Group states that in Britain, 13-14 million people live on half the average income. It goes on to point out that this figure is more than double the number in 1979, with one in three children living in poverty, whilst living standards of the poor and affluent are moving in opposite directions (Oppenheim and Harker 1996).

In 2002 the ONS stated that there were 3.9 million children living in poverty in Britain; this was a reduction of 500,000 since 1997. This still leaves the UK with the highest rate of child poverty in Europe. Child poverty is still defined as any child living in a household with below 60 per cent of average income after housing costs (Batty 2002).

As previously discussed, income alone is an inadequate measure of poverty and its effects. The latest reports (Rahman *et al.* 2001) use a total of 50 indicators to measure poverty and social exclusion. These include income, children living in workless households, low birth weight, births to girls conceiving under age 16, youth unemployment, premature death, obesity, spending on 'essentials', non-participation in civic organisations, lacking a bank account, overcrowding and mortgage arrears. They also outline the trends in each of the indicators, showing changes in the last year and in the medium term. The July 2001 figures show that there were still 13.3 million people living in households with less than 60 per cent of median income. This compared with 13.4 million in 1998-99. Children are likely than average to be in households where there is a low income. Four million children live in households below the threshold, and two million live in workless households. Whilst the number of accidental deaths has halved over the last decade and the number of births to girls under 16 has fallen, the proportion of low birth-weight babies has remained the same. Rates of teenage conception in Britain remain much higher than elsewhere in Western Europe. One in six of the poorest households do not have any type of bank account compared with one in twenty on average incomes. Households with no household insurance are around three times as likely to be burgled as those with insurance. Finally people in low-income households are twice as likely to report that their quality of life is significantly affected by fear of crime than the average and almost twice as likely to feel very dissatisfied with the area in which they live (Rahman *et al.* 2001).

The authors state:

'As a broad generalisation, the poorest in society appear to be sharing in the general improvements. But, on most indicators, significant inequalities continue to exist, with no sign that these are diminishing' (Rahman *et al.* 2001:6).

Whilst the numbers of children who grow up in poverty increase, there is a need to try to understand why poverty persists.

THEORIES AND EXPLANATIONS FOR THE CAUSES OF POVERTY

Whatever the definitions that are used, it is clear that in the UK poverty persists and has increased in the last decade; it thus becomes important to consider why this is so, why the gap between the richer and poorer has widened so much in the last 15 to 20 years and, subsequently, what aspects of contemporary society have shaped the changes. Townsend (1995) has argued that welfare policy to eradicate poverty can no longer limit itself only to the national arena but must address the connection between the local and the global. The new world order requires social policy to be developed in a global framework.

However, at a basic level, the explanations of poverty tend to be either structural or individual; the blame is said to lie with either 'society' or with the poor themselves. This is a broad debate within the social sciences; do structures or individuals hold the primary locus of significance? Some explanations focus on the broad structural definitions of social reality whilst others consider the experiences of individuals and how they construct their understanding. Giddens (1984) suggests interplay between the two: the social, economic and political contexts structure the lives of individuals to some extent but this is despite the efforts of individuals to define and thus shape their own experience. The feminist poststructural framework would support this. Clearly women are individuals; they act in individual ways but they live within the meanings of the day. The discourses on lone mothers are an example, as are the implicit notions of the deserving and undeserving benefit recipient. Beliefs about the role of women, their function and their contribution to society are important. In this study, the concerns are with the women and how they frame their own identity and experiences but their efforts must be seen in the context of the structures and policies that dictate the nature of the social, political and economic environment.

The view that poverty is the fault of the poor summarises the social pathology or cultural explanations of poverty. Poverty, it is argued, can be explained in terms of the characteristics of the poor and the effects of their environment. It is argued that inadequacy and incompetence are to blame and that the inability to compete effectively, and the inability to raise children to compete, results in the transfer of inequality to the next generation. But as Holman (1978) discusses in his examination of the genetic and psychological causes of poverty, most of those who might appear to have inherited the characteristics associated with poverty do not themselves become poor. Victim blaming is a feature of explanations that focus on the family or the community as the cause of poverty.

It was Oscar Lewis who first suggested a so-called culture of poverty. In his work on Mexican families (1965 and 1968), he suggested there were three inter-related aspects of the culture of poverty: first, a range of values, attitudes and beliefs which are different from the rest of society, together with fatalism, helplessness, dependency and inability to defer gratification; second, a range or form of behaviours which are antisocial or which ignore established norms, e.g. promiscuity, illegitimacy, family violence and non-participation in political, social and community institutions; and third, a set of undesirable living conditions with overcrowding, unemployment, ill health, illiteracy and general deprivation.

The first aspect, the values of the poor, is claimed to shape the actions of the second and third aspects of behaviour and life styles. Lewis argues (1966:51) that individuals immersed in a culture of poverty recognise so-called middle-class values but do not live by them. This approach, the cycle of deprivation or the poverty cycle, was adopted and promoted by Keith Joseph in 1972. He argued that poor families resulted from unstable marriages, poor accommodation and overcrowding, inadequate parenting and lack of occupational skills; in other words, the cause was the inherited characteristic of the individual or the people rather than structures. This culture of poverty argument has been used to explain the persistence of poverty from one generation to another. Undoubtedly children who are born to families living in poverty are more likely to be in poverty in adult life and so a certain cyclical pattern is observable, but the issue to consider is whether this is because of personal failings or the structures of society. On the other hand, this explanation does not explain why the poor became poor in the first place, nor does it explain why some individuals and families manage to escape the culture of poverty.

Class is a very important concept in any analysis of poverty. Whilst there have been many attempts to retreat from class or argue that it is 'an increasingly redundant issue' (Holton and Turner 1994 in Skeggs 1997) it is still important as a means of assessing the effects of poverty on individuals. There are many different definitions of class: it is an analytical device used to make sense of a person's economic position and, in particular, to consider the inequalities that such divisions may generate. Skeggs (1997) states that thinking that class does not matter is only the prerogative of those unaffected by the deprivations and exclusions it produces. Class is firmly connected to debates of respectability, which are important in this research and discussed later.

THE UNDERCLASS DEBATE

The term 'underclass' has been used to describe a group of individuals who are trapped outside and below society, a distinct social class somewhere below the working class and the unemployed and thus excluded from mainstream life. There is a tendency to believe that the 'underclass' is a recent invention, but it is likely that a group living outside mainstream life has existed for some time. Runciman (1990) linked the idea of the underclass to the declining role of employment in the manufacturing industry in the late twentieth century.

In 1990, Charles Murray, writing in the *Sunday Times*, suggested that Britain, like America, was developing an underclass. He believed that it was neither firmly established nor composed mainly of minority ethnic groups but nevertheless he saw that the so-called traditional values such as honesty, family life and hard work were being seriously undermined. In the article, he focused on aspects of behaviour rather than the degree of poverty. He described littered and unkempt homes, men unable to keep a job, drunkenness, badly behaved children and crime. He believed that increasing numbers of children were likely to take on these so-called underclass values and transmit the problem to the next generation. His arguments are closely related to those describing the culture of poverty.

The debate concerning the construction of a marginalised underclass of the dependent poor (Murray 1990, 1994) also focuses upon a specific set of values that are said to be instrumental in creating this group. Murray argues that the underclasses are poor from their own choice, depend on state benefits and carry an underclass culture. This is because they do not want to work, do not want to live in traditional nuclear families and are habitually delinquent and criminal. According to Alcock (1997), these arguments reflect the changing debate on the causes of poverty, which emphasises the faults of the poor themselves and the cultural aspects. New poverty, according to Alcock (1997:27), has come to be seen as the product of new social forces, which have a particularly adverse effect on those who used to be called simply 'unemployed' but who now belong to a separate underclass.

In 1973, Rex argued that some of Britain's black communities were becoming a segregated underclass. The elderly, lone parents, the disabled, the chronically sick and the long-term unemployed share a similar description in Townsend (1979:819). For example, he refers to society's imposition upon the elderly of 'underclass' status. The underclass are characterised by their exclusion from the activities and ways of life of the society in which they live. Frank Field (1989), recently a Labour government minister, argues that the underclass is composed of three groups of people: the long-term unemployed, single parents and the elderly poor. He sees four causes of the emergence of an underclass: the rise in unemployment, the widening class divisions, the exclusion of the poor from rising living standards and a change in public attitudes. He describes the move away from sympathy and altruism towards self-interest and selfishness. Field, then in opposition, argued strongly against the idea that characteristics of the underclass were the causes of the problem.

The counterargument to the culture of poverty argument has been made by Taylor-Gooby and Dale (1981) who believe that there is stronger evidence that the wealthy transmit privilege than the poor inherit poverty. Brynner *et al.* (1997), in a recent ESRC-funded study (Economic and Social Research Council), demonstrated that class is still exerting a powerful influence on progress in the 1990s. They discovered that social class remains an important factor in educational achievement. The study makes a division between three distinct groups: those who are 'getting on, those getting by and those getting nowhere'. The 'getting nowhere' group, according to the researchers, are often dependent on benefit and only intermittently in work, have no qualifications or training skills, live with parents or a parent in a broken relationship, and are anxious, depressed and often ill. The view expressed by the GP in the area where the research took place was that there was a fourth group who could be described as 'getting worse'. The inevitable policy response is one that focuses on individuals rather than structures and seeks to change their attitudes and behaviour; as such, it is merely a variation on the culture of poverty idea.

Green (1998:41) continues his criticism of those who adopt a sympathetic approach and seeks to blame those so-called 'poverty professionals', whose philosophy has been one of equalisation rather than independence, for persistently inflating the numbers of the 'poor' by changing the scope of the definition. His more hostile arguments are that the poor are treated as powerless victims of external forces whose problems can only be treated by large cash transfers. His belief is that the cause is individual rather than structural and that redistribution of wealth is not the answer; the poor should be treated as competent individuals who can escape poverty once their enthusiasm and self-confidence are enlisted. He argues that 'the paramount aim in providing help to people who have fallen on hard times should be to empower them to claim their independence, not render them content to lie down under their difficulties'. The government's widening participation in higher education strategy is an example of such a structural intervention. Children from poorer backgrounds will receive up to £1,400 a year to encourage them to remain in education. The government has a target of 50 per cent of under-30 year olds to be in education by 2010.

COMMUNICATION, TECHNOLOGY AND INFORMATION: NEW CAPITAL?

Lash and Urry (1996) offer another explanation of today's society; in particular they explore the effects of capitalism. They argue that in the two-class (the poor and the wealthy) society of the 1990s, the new lower class suffers from increasing poverty; in the USA, Britain and elsewhere, middle-income groups are becoming scarcer as income distribution increasingly assumes a bimodal pattern (1996:160). They assert that the emergence of a new lower class is associated with the growth of the upper income groups. They do not seek to analyse social structures but 'flows'. The flows are not just of people, but also of ideas, images, technologies and capital in and around social groups. Information, technology and new communication strategies can thus be seen as new forms of capital. Their analysis of the economies of signs and space has been focused on the pattern of these flows and the ways in which such flows 'both subvert endogenously determined social structures and provide the preconditions for heightened reflexivity' (1996:321).

Using the example of Los Angeles they show how restructuration after organised capitalism has its basis in increasingly reflexive social actors and organisations. They also point out that the very institutions of organised capitalism, including the welfare state, are themselves at least partly responsible for its eventual disorganisation. Contemporary society is changing rapidly, it is not static, and according to Lash and Urry (1996:165) the new reflexive worlds of today's economies are increasingly economies of sign and space where the subjects are more mobile. Their analysis of changes in social relationships is through the organisation of work, the formation of an underclass and new citizenship. They analyse increasing polarisation with income differentials increasing enormously with a capital-intensive self-service society dependent upon household appliances and leisure services.

They describe the advanced-services middle classes providing a market for each other and for the casualised labour of the new lower class.

The widening gap between the rich and poor must be seen in the context of economic and social change that includes the internationalisation of capital, the decline in manual work, the shift to a service economy and the higher employment of women on generally lower wages. Lash and Urry (1996:323) refer to the end of organised capitalism and describe disordered capitalism as an epoch in which various processes and flows have transformed the previously organised capitalist societies of the north Atlantic rim. They state that the processes and flows which have ushered in such a disorganised capitalism include the following: the flowing of capital and technologies to 170 or so individual 'self governing' capitalist countries, each concerned to defend 'its' territory; time-space compression in financial markets and the development of global cities; the growth in importance of internationalised producer services, the generation of risks, and the punitive globalisation of culture and communication; huge increases in personal mobility of tourists, migrants and refugees; and the development of cosmopolitan tastes for 'fashionable' consumer services. They argue that classes in the hierarchical sense are rapidly dissolving at the same time that social and spatial inequalities are rapidly increasing.

Anthony Giddens (1999) describes the effects of globalisation as emancipation, anxiety, escape from 'fate' and lives fuelled by new sorts of uncertainties. The evidence is in the increase in treaties between sovereign states, links between political parties and trade unions, international business organisations, the growth in arms sales, military interdependence, ethnic diversity, electronic communication, the internet, and a range of other economic and environmental factors. The notion of a 'runaway', out of control society, Giddens argues, needs more not less government and he sees sexual equality as a core principle of democracy (Giddens 1999). The role of women in the new century is seen as crucial.

CURRENT POLICY DEBATES: THE SEARCH FOR STRUCTURAL SOLUTIONS

In 1997, New Labour was elected with a large majority. In a pamphlet published by the Fabian Society (Blair 1998), Tony Blair describes the 'Third Way'. This 'New Politics for the New Century' sets out the ideas, goals and values of the new government. It claims to be based on values such as democracy, liberty, justice, mutual obligation and internationalism. It is described as the Third Way because it moves away from the old Left policies of state control, high taxation and producer interests. It claims to reconcile themes such as rights and responsibilities, as well as promote enterprise and attack poverty and discrimination. There are ambitious targets, including the abolition of child poverty within 20 years.

However, as of 1999-2000, the numbers on low incomes remained at a historic high. Rahman *et al.* (2001) state that in 1999-2000 there were 13.3 million people living with less than 60 per cent of median income (after housing costs). They also state that London has the highest proportion of poor people of any region in England, but also the highest proportion of rich people. Children continue to be more likely to live in low-income households, with 4 million children living in households below the 60 per cent threshold, and 2 million living in workless households. There are energetic structural plans and solutions. These include 'New Deals for Communities': with a budget of £800 million, the aims are to regenerate deprived areas through improving job prospects, reducing crime, improving educational achievement and reducing poor health. There are plans for the government to work in partnership with local authorities, the voluntary sector, business and individuals. An ambitious programme to deal with teenage pregnancy and provide education and training for 16-18 year olds is also on the agenda. The Social Exclusion Unit, reporting directly to the Prime Minister, is charged to produce 'joined up solutions to joined up problems'. The government has a clear aim, constrained by electability, to produce a fairer society; it seeks to change the ways in which both wealth and opportunity are distributed. Central to the government's strategy is action on both the causes and effects of poverty: poor housing, poor health, poor education and a lack of job opportunities are being tackled.

Baroness Jay of Paddington (1999), writing in the *Guardian*, lists the government's policies designed to help women:

'working families tax credit, national minimum wage, the biggest ever increase in child benefit, the guarantee of a nursery place for every four year old, the Sure Start Programme providing for children in vulnerable areas, New Deal for lone parents, child care tax credit to help families on low incomes, parental leave, family emergency leave, enhanced employment rights, measures to fight violence against women and support for carers' (Jay 1999).

This is an impressive list and favours those in employment but does little for the women in this study who are living in poverty.

Women find themselves in a contradictory position in New Labour's policy and rhetoric. As we have seen, women find themselves living in poverty for a variety of reasons. Women are either dependent on men, dependent on state benefits or employed in areas where they are traditionally paid less than men. Women are over-represented amongst the ranks of low-paid workers. Women's work as mothers and carers is still not recognised, neither is their vulnerability to poverty within families. Apart from increases in child benefit, paid directly to women, they will benefit little from the government's policies. A nursery education at four years of age will not help them find employment in the first four years of their child's life. The assumption that women live in families, dependent on men, supported by men, dominates the government's thinking. The public discourses about the family are powerful and dominant. Marriage and parenting are seen as the foundations of family life and by implication the basics of 'good society'. It is women's unpaid labour that allows men to earn more. Women's position in the world of New Labour is still tied to notions of the deserving and the undeserving poor. Because women are still seen as dependents of men, their rights to welfare provision and state benefits are constantly challenged. Women on benefits are seen as a 'problem' to be solved. Whilst the deserving poor, such as the elderly and widows, have rights, the undeserving, single women with children have duties and responsibilities. Good women should be at home, being financially supported by men. If the men are low-wage earners, then they will be offered a range of enhanced benefits provided by the government. These policies assume that all women are the same and offer solutions that are unrelated to individual experiences and the realities of their lives.

The tensions in the Third Way proposals revolve around the expectation that women will work. Not only is a woman expected to live with a man whose duty is to provide for her but in order to resolve the problem of her poverty she will move from 'welfare to work'. At the same time, there is no available child-care provision for children under four years of age or during school holidays and no well-paid jobs for women. There is also an assumption that 'communities' as such exist and can be galvanised into action on the range of problems highlighted by the government. It is believed that universal problems demand universal solutions, which ignore the individual experience of women.

These so-called Third Way policies are complex; there are a significant number of social programmes including health action zones, education action zones, new deals for communities and the Social Exclusion Unit. As well as the special projects, the government action on poverty has led to the minimum wage, a higher working families tax credit, higher pensions for the poorest, new child-care tax credits and significant increases in child benefit. Polly Toynbee also believes that simply increasing benefits is insufficient. She argues in the *Guardian* (1999:19) that benefits alone will never produce the massive shift in opportunity and wealth towards the poor. Getting the poorest into work and paying good in-work subsidies are essential. Toynbee reiterates the key message of poverty campaigners: 'children are poor because their mothers are poor and many more children are now poorer than twenty years ago largely because they depend on their mother's incomes alone and mothers of poor children earn far too little'. The pay gap between women's and men's earnings is a crucial issue in poverty research and it contributes significantly to child poverty.

An integral part of the Third Way policies is the system of paying benefits. This has always been a contentious issue. Alistair Darling (1999), who at the time of writing was the Social Security Secretary, believes that simply increasing benefits is insufficient and reiterates the government's line of 'work for those who can, security for those who cannot'. The aim is to encourage welfare claimants to take work. In 1988, Margaret Thatcher, the then Prime Minister, spoke of the apparent problem of young, single girls who were deliberately getting pregnant in order to jump the housing queue and obtain benefits (*Guardian* 23 November 1988). The ideas were reinforced during the 1993 election campaign when a series of attacks on single mothers was made. Welfare benefits and housing, it was argued, should only be available to 'respectable, married women'; indeed the provision of benefits might actually act as an incentive to young women to become pregnant. Women as single mothers have been constructed as deviant, destructive forces in society, and an underclass. The lone mother is the subject of public anxiety and moral panics and seen as unnatural and a problem to be solved. The traditional heterosexual family is seen as central, normal, natural and as such the most desirable.

Various solutions to women's poverty have been suggested. One overly simple suggestion is that women should not be paid benefits at all but should work, although the work available is low paid and difficult. Bradshaw *et al.* (1996), in a study funded by the Joseph Rowntree Foundation, stated that the United Kingdom has one of the highest proportions of lone-parent families in the European Union and the lowest rate of employment. Working as a way out of poverty is unrealistic in a society where the high cost of child care creates a strong disincentive to work and where child care is only provided for vulnerable and at-risk children. The housing benefit system, paid to all the women in this study, is another major factor. When women work, they no longer receive income support and lose housing benefit. Bradshaw et al. argue that child care must be affordable, and available after school and in school holidays, if women are to return to work. This report fails to acknowledge that for some women, staying with their children may also be an acceptable option. For the women in this study, paid employment was an unrealistic option; having a child or children to care for was enough. They were caught in a classic poverty trap. If they took the low-paid factory work that was readily available they would lose out on housing benefit, free school meals for their other children and still have to find the cost of child care. All the women involved in this study were convinced that their work was child care; this was their priority and the main reason for their life. Occasionally they were disturbed by reports on the government's Welfare to Work programme but they remained convinced that no government, especially a Labour government, would force them to go out to work when they were either pregnant or the mothers of children under five.

SOCIAL EXCLUSION

Social exclusion is a term first used in France, adopted by the European Union and later used by the New Labour government. It is a relatively new term in British policy and refers not only to poverty and low income but also to some of the wider causes and consequences. Batty (2002) argues that the government has defined social exclusion as 'what can happen when people or areas suffer from a combination of linked problems such as unemployment, poor skills, low income, poor housing, high crime, bad health and family breakdown' (*Guardian* 15 January 2002). According to Ruth Lister (1999), it is more than a euphemism for poverty; it is a multidimensional concept embracing a variety of ways in which people are denied full participation in society and full effective rights of citizenship in the civil, political and social spheres. There is a danger that if the term is used uncritically it can obscure poverty. Traditionally the Labour Party's policies have reflected the need to redistribute income and wealth principally through the income tax system. Nevertheless, after 18 years in opposition, the Blair government's strategy for reforming welfare can be cautiously welcomed. The Thatcher years were dominated by a Right-leading agenda, which did little to address the multiple problems of women and poverty.

At the 1997 Labour Party Conference, Tony Blair said, 'a decent society is not based on rights. It is based on our duty to each other. The new welfare system must encourage work, not dependency'. He was unclear as to how women fitted in to the new vision; were women to stay at home in families, care for their children and be supported by men earning a decent wage or were they to go out and join the labour market and contribute to the family? He went on to set out the need for the long-term unemployed and the young to take up options that are part of the investment in welfare and training. He said that single mothers must at least visit a job centre and not 'just stay at home waiting for a benefit cheque every week until the children are sixteen'. He did not explain the arrangements for child care at this stage.

In 1998, the government set up the Social Exclusion Unit. In the supporting literature the definition of social exclusion draws upon that provided by Batty (2002); social exclusion is defined as 'a shorthand label for what can happen when individuals or areas suffer from a combination of linked problems such as unemployment, poor skills, low incomes, poor housing, high crime environments, bad health and family breakdown'. The literature claims that although the government has policies that are targeting each of these aspects individually, the government has been less successful in tackling the interaction between problems and preventing such problems arising in the first place.

In *Social Trends* 32 (ONS 2002) social exclusion is further elaborated:

'Being disadvantaged, and thus "excluded" from many of the opportunities available to the average citizen, has often been seen as synonymous with having a low income. While low income is clearly central to poverty and social exclusion, it is now widely accepted that there is a wide range of other factors that are important. People can experience poverty of education, of training, of health and of environment as well as poverty in purely cash terms' (2002:98).

The structural responses to these complex and multidimensional problems include the initiatives such as the Social Exclusion Unit and health and education action zones.

The purpose of the Social Exclusion Unit, chaired by the Prime Minister himself, is to improve understanding of the key characteristics of social exclusion and promote solutions. The priority tasks are truancy and school exclusions, street living or homelessness and what are described as 'Worst Estates'. The task is to develop integrated and sustainable approaches to the problems of worst housing estates including crime, community breakdown, bad schools etc. In its first phase, the unit will focus on drawing up key indicators of social exclusion and recommend how these can be tracked to monitor the effectiveness of government policies. Whitehall units for neighbourhood renewal, rough sleepers, teenage pregnancy, and children and young people to improve joint working have been set up.

According to the government's own figures these units have proved effective in tackling social exclusion. The Social Exclusion Unit is part of a wider government effort to tackle social inclusion; the Sure Start programmes launched in 1998 co-ordinate programmes to improve the health and well-being of pre-school children in deprived areas. Many midwives have found new roles working as part of these schemes.

Ruth Lister in the Annual Lecture on Social Change, Birmingham (1999), said 'inclusion into the bottom rung of an unequal society in which the rich are able to exclude themselves from common bonds of citizenship is a less than inspiring vision'. She argued that whilst paid work was important it did not necessarily spell genuine social inclusion for those trapped in dead-end jobs. It also undervalues other forms of work such as community and voluntary work and the work of many women, that of unpaid work in the home. As ever, women living in poverty with children, married and unmarried, are firmly on the bottom rung on a very unequal society.

According to O'Brian and Penna (1998:3) social welfare policies and systems – in one view, the cure for poverty – are embedded in visions of a 'good society' and each proposal for or understanding of social welfare is inextricably linked with a wider analysis of social life. They argue that 'theory is a dimension of action in so far as it gives direction and meaning to what we do'. Theories are generalisations about what exists in the world around us and how the components of that world fit together into patterns. They suggest that theories are 'abstractions' in that they generalise across situations, expectations and suppositions about the reasons why patterns exist and how we should deal with them. O'Brian and Penna (1998) believe that it is necessary not only to be aware of theories and assumptions that shape social policy but also to recognise that it is different theories that enable individuals to see the effects and consequences of policies. They argue that some social theories of welfare reject the focus on the welfare state altogether, emphasising the patterns of cultural and social division that maintain inequality and disadvantage both within and outside the formal institutions of welfare state services. The focus of this theory is on struggles and conflicts that sustain the hierarchical relations between different groups. The role of the state in providing resources is a dimension of the struggle, not a cause or response to disadvantage.

In this chapter I have debated some of the complexities that surround the definition and measurement of poverty. I have considered the incidence and extent of poverty in the United Kingdom and some of the theories and explanations for the causes of poverty. I have considered the underclass debate and returned to the government's proposed solutions as set out in the Third Way proposals. I have briefly discussed the tensions and contradictions that surround the issues of welfare benefits and the pressure on childbearing women to work. In the next chapter I will describe how I gathered the data for the study.

3

Gathering the data

INTRODUCTION

This chapter describes the methodology that I used in this study. It describes the research process; the methodological issues and debates are considered in relation to each stage in the story of the research process. I begin by describing various epistemological positions and explain how a framework of feminist poststructuralism has guided the research and the data collection. I consider the various definitions of ethnography and the debates that inform the use of qualitative data. I describe the process of obtaining ethical approval and debate some of the ethical issues that are important in conducting research on and with women. I analyse the process of negotiating access, the choice of the sample and the various methods that I used to gather data. In this chapter, I have also explored some aspects of the impact of the research on the researcher. I discuss the process of analysis and some of the pleasures and difficulties of the fieldwork. I debate the use of interviews as a data collection tool and consider the issues and tensions around bias, objectivity, reliability, validity, and trustworthiness in ethnographic research.

This research is a feminist ethnography. It is concerned with women and women's lives. It is placed in a feminist poststructural framework. One of the key areas of feminist poststructural thought is the concern with the difficulties of only producing a partial story of women's lives. Olesen (2000) argues that, for poststructuralists, truth is a destructive illusion and knowledge is always partial and limited. The emphasis here is on fluid conceptions of women's experiences with consideration of discourse, narrative and text. In this research, it is recognised that experience is individual and cannot be generalised and that the search for meaning, like the search for truth, is ongoing. With these limitations I wanted to explore the experiences of this group of women; I recognised that I was working with individual women with individual and different experiences.

Sandra Harding, a philosopher, recognised three types of feminist enquiry, which she termed 'transitional epistemologies' (Harding 1987:186). Feminist empiricism was divided into two types: *spontaneous feminist empiricism*, with rigorous adherence to existing research norms and standards, and *contextual empiricism* which recognises the social values and interest of science. The third, *standpoint theory*, claims that all knowledge attempts are socially situated and that some of these objective social locations are better than others for knowledge projects. Postmodern theories void the possibility of a feminist science in favour of the many and multiple stories that women tell. It was Harding's concern with feminist research as a scientific activity and the attempt to generate 'less false stories' that prompted her reliance on processes strictly governed by methodological rules. She argued that researchers should examine critically their own personal and historical commitments with which they construct their work (Harding 1987:70). Harding argues for 'strong objectivity', which contrasts sharply with value-free objectivity. I will return to Harding's work on 'strong objectivity' later in this chapter. Harding's work is important in challenging assumptions of objectivity but the framework that drives this research is one of feminist poststructuralism and its refusal to acknowledge that there can be universalised and normalising accounts of women as a group, that assumptions of a shared singular identity should be challenged and that meaning is only ever partial and incomplete. I recognised that whatever efforts I made and however rigorous my methods and techniques I could only ever know part of the story. I believed that, even in part, an incomplete story was still worth hearing.

DEFINING ETHNOGRAPHY

In order to investigate the lives of a marginalised group (childbearing women living in poverty), I chose ethnography. I felt that there could be no other method or approach that would enable me to study the lives of women and listen to their own stories. The result, this ethnography, is based on two years of fieldwork, working closely with childbearing women and their families. All the women were in receipt of means-tested benefits; by all the standard definitions, they were childbearing women living in poverty in the West Midlands at the end of the twentieth century.

Ethnography is qualitative research; it uses observation, analysis of texts and documents, interviews, transcribing, field notes and what are sometimes described as 'hanging about', 'sussing out', listening and thinking. The approaches to feminist research are highly diversified and have developed rapidly during the last 25 years. Ethnographic research like all other research has to be rigorous, systematic, organised and purposeful.

Olesen (2000) has argued that 'rage is not enough' and has called for incisive scholarship to frame, direct and harness passions in the interests of redressing grievous problems in many areas of women's health and lives. In the growing complexity, fundamental questions such as whose knowledge, where and how is it obtained, by whom, from whom and for what purposes have to be addressed. The writings from women of colour, queer theorists and women with disabilities have all challenged the grounds and process of doing feminist research. The key concepts of experience, difference and gender are under scrutiny as are aspects such as the role of the researcher and her ability to be an all-knowing, distanced, context-free seeker of objectified knowledge whose gender in some way guarantees access to women's lives and knowledge. It is in considering these assumptions that researchers should examine their own position and attributes and the impact of the research on both the researcher and the researched. In the Introduction, I have attempted to describe my own motivations for the research and my own trajectory from working-class to middle-class researcher.

Atkinson (1990) describes the ethnographer as constructing versions of social reality and engaging in the task of persuading the reader of its authenticity, plausibility and significance. The data, from which the published text is derived, are constructed and consist of authored representations of social scenes. Atkinson argues that there is a process of translation and transcription that goes through many stages in the creation of the narratives. This book is the result of that process of translation. The narratives presented in the later chapters are the result of thought, intuition, interpretation and analysis.

Lareau and Shultz (1996) say that reasonable people disagree about the definition of ethnography. It can include the use of participant observation to study a community for an extended period. It is a holistic approach and includes the portrayal of a community from the perspective of the participants. It can be a focus on culture and a focus on context. Almost all definitions include the use of participant observations as well as in-depth interviews with key informants. There is almost always a need to be in the setting long enough to acquire some notion of acceptance and understanding. It is a complex yet simple research method.

Ethnographic research takes place in a natural setting. It makes use of human skills such as sensitivity, compassion, intuition, concern and, in my case, was partially motivated by anger at inequality and a desire for justice and equity. The tools of the ethnographer are watching, listening, asking questions, interviewing, note taking, and the review of diaries, life histories and other documents; then thinking and analysing the views, feelings, attitudes, beliefs and values of the people. The initial task, therefore, was to observe, describe and explain. Ethnography stresses the importance of studying human behaviour in the context of a culture, and the aim is to understand aspects of that culture, so as to uncover its rules, values and norms.

According to Hammersley and Atkinson (1995), the primary aim should be to describe what happens in the setting: how the people involved see their own actions and those of others, as well as describing the context in which those actions take place. These writers, with others, also emphasise the importance of the researcher having respect and appreciation of the social world being studied. It is the business of ethnography to discover the shape and limits of social systems and cultural worlds. In the ethnographic process, these discoveries unfold gradually as the fieldwork proceeds, rather than their parameters being set in advance. Rather than studying people, the ethnographer seeks to learn from people, to grasp the emic or the 'natives' point of view. According to Hammersley and Atkinson:

'The ethnographer participates in people's daily lives for an extended period of time, watching what happens, listening to what is said, asking questions, in fact, collecting whatever data are available to throw light on the issues that are the focus of the research' (1995:1).

In this study, the data were collected over a two-year period and, although the starting point was an exploration of women's experiences of childbirth, other issues became more prominent and significant during the fieldwork. Ethnography has also been described as the study of culture; culture consists of the rules that generate and guide behaviour. Leininger (1985) has been at the leading edge in nursing research, using this method, and describes ethnography as:

'The systematic process of observing, detailing, describing, documenting and analysing the lifeways or particular patterns of a culture (or subculture), in order to grasp the lifeways or patterns of people in their familiar environment.'

Agar (1986) describes ethnography as the process of encountering an alien world and trying to explain it. He suggests that the purpose is to learn about a world that is not understood by encountering it first-hand and making sense out of it. This requires intensive personal involvement, an improvisational style, and the ability to learn from mistakes. In this study, the world was sometimes alien, sometimes familiar, and the coping strategies which were adopted innovative and at times surprising. Agar's description of ethnography is that it is neither objective nor subjective, but interpretative, mediating two worlds through a third. The qualitative data that emerged from the study needed to be interpreted and explained.

Ethnography has its philosophical basis in the value of culture, naturalism and holism. Many qualitative philosophies and research traditions argue that the complex social world in which individuals live and operate cannot be understood in terms of simple cause and effect relationships. The method is based on the belief that human action is complex – informed by social meanings, influenced by intentions, values, rules, beliefs and aspects of culture – and as such cannot be understood only in terms of scientific laws. Although ethnography can be used to test theories, this study is not directed to this goal. It does, however, aim to refine and develop understanding of pre-existing theory. It seeks to provide concrete descriptions and will include the process of analytic deduction. The purpose is not only to determine the tactics individuals adopt to make sense of their experiences, but also to try to understand these strategies and actions as part of the whole, and as part of the society in which women live.

Hammersley and Atkinson (1995) emphasise the importance of the researcher having respect and appreciation of the social world being studied. Hobbs and May (1993) are concerned with how to establish 'closeness' and 'authenticity' in social scientific accounts of other people's lives. In 'telling it like it is' and from the inside the researcher is required to be both on the inside as a researcher and on the outside as one who communicates the story to the outside world. This was very difficult but not impossible to achieve. The work was challenging yet absorbing and fulfilling.

Jocelyn Cornwall, writing in 1984, chose the ethnographic method as the most appropriate way of investigating people's lives as a whole. She argues that the ethnographic approach is one that encourages attention to the detail of people's lives and thus to the differences between individuals:

'This approach makes it more rather than less likely that interpretations of ethnographic material will bear witness to the part each person plays in shaping the course of his or her own life without losing sight of the fact that they do so in conditions that are not of their own choosing' (1984:204).

Her defence of the ethnographic method is well described and she concludes that only by using repeated interviews with the same families and by establishing relationships with those she studied was she able to gain the information and understanding that she did.

Recently, ethnography has been subjected to a very critical reassessment. The value of fieldwork has been confirmed but, according to Silverman (1998), the focus is now on demonstrating the relationship between forms and heterogeneous action, rather than trying to identify a culture as a whole. There is now a need to understand the complexity of action, to gain access to the collective wholes that govern behaviour. Silverman argues that, in the past, it was sufficient to observe, describe, explain and understand. Now it is necessary to aggregate, or bring together, and contextualise observations and this is what I tried to do in the study. There is still a need for an empirical approach; there is still a need to remain open to elements that cannot be codified and a concern for grounding the phenomena observed in the field. An ethnographic study is a study of human activities, in all its forms; it has an empirical approach, there must be an openness of observation, and it must happen in the natural setting. The study must be grounded in the specific historical and cultural context, and to be a feminist ethnography, the work must matter to women. It is a qualitative, descriptive work that seeks to understand aspects of culture and the nature of individuals' experiences. The methods include in-depth interviewing and participant and non-participant observation. When searching for the collective whole, the ethnographer must avoid the trap of defining a universal experience and the further trap of offering universal solutions.

Authenticity, rather than reliability, is the issue in qualitative research, the aim being to produce an authentic understanding of people's experiences. In this study, I asked women to tell me what they saw as their story. I recognise that those stories are individual and are based on that person's own experiences and are shaped by the values and beliefs of those around her and who have influenced her. Merely focusing on women's experience does not take into account how those experiences have emerged and what the material, historical and social circumstances were. Each woman was unique. She had a unique past, a unique set of beliefs and values and a unique set of family, friends and acquaintances.

According to O'Leary (1997:47), personal experience is not a self-authenticating claim to knowledge; there is a danger of essentialism in unthinking reliance on experience. Olesen (2000) refers to Joan Scott who aptly comments: 'Experience is at once already an interpretation and in need of interpretation.'

Armed with this knowledge and at times with great uncertainty as to the value of my work, I used a tape recorder to provide a record of the interaction and conversations with women. I aimed to gather information, first-hand, in a natural setting. I worked in women's homes, in the GP surgery, in the community office, in the job centre, in the antenatal clinic, in the playground, in the local supermarket, the chemist and the Oxfam shop. The community midwives arranged the visits and often took me to the women's homes. Transcripts of informal conversations and interviews were compared with field notes. I transcribed all the interviews that I could and I kept a reflective diary and detailed field notes.

As previously explained, obtaining interview data was often difficult. Standard interview texts advise a quiet room without interruptions. The reality was very different. Sometimes the noise from the television, and from the other children present, drowned out the recordings. Often the mothers and sisters of the women I spoke to stayed and joined in the interview. Conversation, talk and chat provided the raw data of ethnographic research. The voices of men were absent from the study; I openly invited them to stay and talk, but the women would send them away or they would get up and walk out. Some said that they had no part in 'women's business'; others looked uncomfortable and walked away. The majority were absent anyway.

Childbearing women living in poverty traditionally do not contribute to information-gathering exercises; they do not respond to surveys. As I have explained earlier it was also impossible to gain access to the local Bengali community or to obtain permission to speak with women from other black and minority ethnic communities who were also living in poverty and accessing the maternity services. The experiences of this group, women living in poverty, still require empirical observation. There is still a need to remain open, and to discover the elements that make up everyday life. There is still a need to consider how people interact with others, and the world in which they find themselves. The unexpected elements must still be allowed to reveal themselves; there must still be openness, flexibility, reflexivity and compassion (Silverman 1998).

A study becomes ethnographic when the field worker connects what she sees is happening – in this case, the issues and passions of childbearing women living in poverty – to the backdrop against which these happenings occur; happenings are both historical and cultural. There is a clear need to ask the questions: why are these women living in this way, and what forces and actions have occurred to make them live and act in the way that they do, in this time and this place? Why is there poverty in the West Midlands, and why do these women appear to bear the brunt of poverty in the way that they do?

As described by Silverman (1993), ethnography is empirical, open, embedded in a field and the science of the particular. A series of ethnographic studies, such as this, can serve as sources for defining the universal human phenomena in a true sense. In a true ethnographic study, the researcher feels, touches, smells, lives, shops and thinks in the field, and then relates the whole to the global referential framework. It involves empathy, immersion in the field and gaining access to the point of view of others, in an attempt to understand that world. The researcher has to separate mentally and physically from her familiar universe, and be physically present in the new environment. Understanding of the cultural whole is achieved by making sense out of what is seen, heard and talked about.

In practical terms, it means working your way through the dense fabric of the culture, in order to arrive at an understanding of issues. This has included examining the social order of shopping, exploring the complexities of relationships, and the deeply held views about the values of having children. It has meant being part of the planning for the pending arrival of the bailiffs and watching as a woman's worldly goods and chattels are bundled into the loft and eased through a hole in the wall to the neighbour's property to outwit the bailiff and prevent seizure of goods. It has meant poring over the contract for the Sky digital television and being part of the ceremonial order of the benefits office. It has involved watching the fight with the housing department, the encounter with the loan shark, the debates with the drug dealer, the aftermath of physical assault, the tactics for sidestepping the health visitor or for negotiation and communication with the police and much more. It has been an intensely emotional experience and often exhausting. It is integrative ethnography and an attempt to relate sequences of ethnographic tradition to the cultural whole.

Silverman (1998) has argued that, for many years, it has been the development of theory that has provided the impetus for research; theories are developed and modified by good research, but he also warns researchers against accepting, uncritically, the conventional wisdoms of the day. Such wisdoms often suggest that childbearing women living in poverty are all feckless, irresponsible, deeply unhappy, stressed and are out to only exploit the social security system. Conventional wisdom ignores the individual and the individual's responses to the challenges of life. Similarly, theories imply that the truth is out there to be found and it is only through 'good' research that the truth can be found. Silverman warns the qualitative researcher against being a 'tourist'. Research 'tourists' begin without a hypothesis, gaze rapaciously at social scenes, and focus on groups and subgroups so intently that they fail to recognise similarities between their own cultures and those they are studying. He also warns against romanticism; the researcher carefully and faithfully records the 'experiences' of childbearing women living in poverty, but can easily neglect to recognise how 'experience' itself is shaped by cultural forms of representation. Explanations offered by women about the men in their lives may be simply a culturally given way of understanding, accepting and explaining the actions of their partners. The explanations offered by women themselves are compared with the views held by their grandmothers and other relatives. The aim is to understand more of how things are, and more of why they might be as they are.

Silverman also calls for historic sensitivity, that is, looking at the relevant historical evidence. In this study, the questions are many and varied but include asking: how did this country come to have so many women and children living in poverty? What policies and events have resulted in the gap between the rich and the poor becoming so wide in recent years? And why is there still poverty in the late 1990s and early twenty-first century? Silverman calls for political sensitivity, encouraging researchers to ask why 'political problems' became defined as such. Why is the government of today concerned about the plight of the poor and the increase in teenage pregnancy? Is it compassion, a belief in a fair and just society, or simply a matter of cost? The feminist perspective on the research also must relate the political definitions of problems to the position of women, and in particular childbearing women, living in poverty in this society. There is no single answer to these questions: just as there are multiple determinants of problems, there are multiple explanations and understandings. The meaning changes and develops as knowledge and understanding develops.

Contextual sensitivity requires the researcher to recognise that uniform institutions, such as the family, take on a variety of meanings in different contexts, and that childbearing women in poverty produce a context for what they do in their own lives. Researchers should not simply import their own assumptions as to what is significant or relevant in any context. Over-interpretation and simple description can lead to inaccurate assumptions. Any ethnographic study must be grounded in its specific cultural context.

BEING PART OF THE CULTURE

During the research period, I lived in the locality, approximately one mile from the housing estate where most of the data were gathered. I had moved to the West Midlands as part of my work and I had bought a new house on an upmarket, modern estate. My children did not attend the local schools; my assessment of the league tables persuaded me to enrol them at other schools some distance away. I never really felt part of the area; I always felt like an incomer and despite my attempts to engage with my neighbours I always felt on the outside. Despite this, I shopped at the same shops, attended the same local events and shared the local GP. In many senses, I lived in the field, but I remained an outsider; I was seen as different by my neighbours. I had spent most of my adult life in Wales and although I have lived in the West Midlands for the past four years I had not acquired a Black Country accent. Despite this uncomfortable background, I tried to bring my skills as a midwife, empathy, compassion and an interest in their lives. I found the fieldwork uncomfortable, tense and difficult.

GETTING STARTED: THE ETHICS COMMITTEE

Apart from the formalities of writing a research proposal and registering at a university, my key task was to secure local health authority ethics committee approval, and to negotiate access to the research site and to the women and the families that I wanted to meet. I approached the Walsall Health Authority Ethics Committee and submitted a research proposal, a series of information sheets and consent forms. These included: a community midwife explanatory letter, information form and consent form; an information sheet for women participating in the study; a consent form for women and their partners; and a GP information letter and consent form. The responses of the committee, used to dealing with requests to undertake drug trials and double-blind controlled trials of various treatments, were detailed and required significant additional information. The main issues that were raised were presented as questions and prerequisites to them granting permission. The questions/comments were:

1. Although the interviews may not be structured, we require greater details of what topics will be covered in the interviews.
2. The fact that interviews may be taped should be made more explicit on the information sheets.
3. The letter to GPs should not require them to opt out, but to opt in to the recruitment of individuals. GPs should be provided with a stamped addressed envelope and give his [sic] clear consent for you to speak to his [sic] patients on each occasion.
4. The General Medical Council guidelines on handling tape recordings should be followed.
5. If the interview is likely to cover sensitive or potentially embarrassing topics, some reference should be given in the information sheet.
6. The committee expresses concern as to how the researcher might 'ascertain the patient's social status'.
7. Please clarify the role of the community midwife.

8. If access to medical records is required, patient and doctor written consent must be obtained.

I was able to comply with all of the above requirements, and answer the questions, and eventually permission to undertake the study was granted. The medical profession which controls such committees operates from a positivist and very structuralist perspective. It was difficult but not impossible to negotiate the access I required.

ETHNOGRAPHY: A FEMINIST METHODOLOGY?

Feminist research such as this is has been described as being on women, *for* and *with* women and in this case conducted by a woman. Research *for* women tries to take into account women's needs, interests and experiences and aims to improve women's lives in one way or another. Wilkinson (1986) believes that feminist research is research *on* women, and *for* women, 'giving priority to female experience and developing theory which is firmly situated in this experience'. Wise (1987), a radical feminist, takes a stronger line and suggests that feminist research should be 'concerned with women's oppression and should be located within a model where the power imbalance (between researcher and researched) can be broken down'. Such assertions assume that all women are oppressed, all women are victims of an imbalance of power and all are vulnerable. Bernhard (1984) suggests eight criteria for feminist research which, though rather dated, are helpful in guiding the research process. These are:

1. The researcher is a woman.
2. Feminist methodology is used including subject interaction, non-hierarchical research relationships, expressions of feelings and concern for values.
3. The research has the potential to help its subjects.
4. The focus is on the experiences of women.
5. It is a study of women.
6. The words 'feminism' or 'feminist' are actually used (this is now out of date, and the use of these terms in not always necessary).
7. Feminist literature is cited.
8. The research is reported using non-sexist language.

Using these criteria as my guide, but constantly acknowledging that women are individuals and not a homogeneous group, I set about the study.

Stacey (1988) argues that ethnography is not always beneficial; it can be exploitative. Women who are researched are also subjected to other risks. They are vulnerable and at risk of inadvertent exploitation and misrepresentation. There is the risk of patronising and offending the subjects of the research, there is a risk of misunderstanding and misinterpreting their lives and there is the even bigger risk of making their lives worse as I explore, probe, uncover and then walk away. The ethical dilemmas are about power and the abuse of power: when women talk to me willingly and openly, they give me even more power and this has to be recognised and acknowledged. I was acutely aware of the balance of power throughout the data-collection stages of the study.

In the early days of feminist research, it was argued that there should always be non-hierarchical relations between the researcher and the researched, but this is naive. How can I, a middle-class, professional woman, claim to be equal to those who live in poverty in the West Midlands? How can I pretend that we will both gain equally from my research? I recognised that an imbalance of power probably existed. Olesen (2000) cites the work of Ong (1995) who has argued that feminist qualitative researchers have looked more closely at the relations that develop between researchers and participants. The image of the powerless respondent has altered with the recognition that the researcher's 'power is often only partial, illusory, tenuous and confused with the researcher responsibility'; this is despite the fact that researchers may be more powerfully positioned when out of the field, because they will write the accounts.

I respected the rights of the women who chose to speak with me and the rights of those who chose not to or opted out at some stage. I followed the Department of Health and Royal College of Nursing guidelines on confidentiality and storage of data. I also worked on the principle that gaining consent was an ongoing process. When I was treated as an 'insider', and allowed to share women's confidences, it was even more important to ensure that their informed consent was still being given. The basic ethical principles of beneficence, to try to do good, and non-maleficence, to minimise harm, guided the process of the research. Issues of privacy, consent, confidentiality and deceit are as important in feminist ethnographic research as in any other area. The research process has to be decent and fair and avoid harm of any sort in the course of data collection, analysis or publication. Other issues that arise in this type of research relate to who owns the data. It could be argued that the women are exploited by the research process; they contribute but the benefits in terms of changing clinical midwifery practice are distant and remote. The benefits to the researcher have the potential to be considerably greater. Olesen (2000) argues that participants are in some ways always 'doing' research; they, along with researchers, construct meanings that become data for interpretation. I was able to identify partially with the participants and was part of their construction of their accounts of their lives.

Ribbens and Edwards (1998) describe social research as a difficult and perplexing task requiring sensitivity on many different levels. In their edited collection they seek to explore the interplay between theory, ways of knowing about the social world, and methodology and practice in qualitative studies. The interplay and tension is explored between the 'private' lives of women in their domestic, intimate and personal lived experiences and the public discussion as the ethnographer communicates her findings to the academic world. Hearing women's voices raises practical problems and challenges and the responsibility to honour the contribution they make. The issues that women raise must be considered, confronted and explored. The researchers cannot sanitise their accounts nor ignore their words. Ribbens and Edwards describe the researcher as 'placed on the edges, between public social knowledge and private lived experience'(1998:2). The researcher makes 'public' the private and personal, and this bringing of private lives into public knowledge is both uncomfortable and difficult. The dilemma of qualitative exploration of the intimate lives of the women of Middleton and the making public of that exploration remains a contentious issue.

All research is beset with dilemmas and difficulties. An ethnographic study of childbearing women in poverty is no exception. There had to be a fundamental belief that what I was doing was good, worthwhile and honourable. I was determined to value and respect this group of women throughout the process.

NEGOTIATING ACCESS

Building on my established position in midwifery, negotiating access with other gatekeepers was relatively simple. I sought an interview with the Director of Nursing, the Head of Midwifery and the Community Midwifery Manager. Without exception, they were enthusiastic, supportive and encouraging.

Despite the optimistic start, I failed completely to gain access to women who lived in predominantly black and minority ethnic communities. All the women I worked with were white. The GPs as gatekeepers in the other areas were distrustful and reluctant to help. I tried to negotiate, to find other ways of listening and talking to other groups of women, but I was unsuccessful. Only one GP actively encouraged and supported my request to conduct the research in the area covered by his practice. Later, at a conference, I met two community midwives who 'worked the patch' and who were prepared to facilitate the fieldwork. This proved to be an invaluable resource and opportunity but sadly in their area there were no women from black or minority ethnic groups. I then spent an interesting week meeting the relevant health professionals and explaining the requirements of the ethics committee. Next I spent time oiling the wheels of the research; I was involved in meeting the practice receptionists, health visitors, district nurses and care attendants and other health-care workers. Without exception, I was welcomed enthusiastically and encouraged to share my findings at the earliest opportunity.

Access to individual women and their families in this particular community was always straightforward and facilitated by the community midwives. In the early days of the study, they made the initial requests on my behalf. They spoke with the women who lived in the area and explained the purpose of the research. This gave the women the opportunity to refuse to take part before ever meeting with me. As the study progressed, and I was known in the area, women themselves sought me out. It became known that I would usually attend the 'Friday clinic', and many women used this opportunity to approach me. The community midwives distributed information sheets and explained verbally to anyone who was interested what the study was about. They also explained that I was a midwife, doing research, and was eager to know their views and listen to their stories. Many women commented that they liked the title, 'Listening to Women', and felt keen to talk to me. Word quickly spread amongst the 'Friday clinic women', and I had no difficulty at all in obtaining the women's permission to undertake the study, or talk to them and their families. If, at any stage, a woman wanted to opt out of the study, this was arranged. Women were not put under pressure to comply or continue with the study. Some women dropped out and then rejoined the study. They did this by contacting me directly, or by leaving a message at the GP surgery or with one of the midwives. On other occasions, they would just not arrive at an agreed interview.

THE SAMPLE

Two principles guided the selection of the sample: appropriateness and adequacy. Appropriateness was derived from identification and utilisation of women who were living in poverty, on state benefits and who were willing and able to spend time talking with me. Adequacy meant that the study continued until there was sufficient data to provide the full and rich descriptions that were required. I also reached what is sometimes described as saturation, when the data becomes repetitive and no new areas emerge. The sample was a convenience sample, selected from women who were pregnant during 1998-99, and registered with the GP at the local surgery and living in the same geographical area. The women were not randomly selected and therefore cannot be regarded as 'typical' or 'representative' in the statistical sense. They were individuals who were willing to give me some time and who were willing to talk to me. Overall, 25 women contributed to the study. All were living in poor quality local authority housing, in run-down areas, and were in receipt of means-tested benefits. A brief profile of the main respondents is included in 'Introducing the Women'. The average age was 23; eleven were single, four described themselves as cohabiting, four were married and six were divorced. It was found that around one third had had a miscarriage and two thirds had experienced ill health in the previous year. In addition, two thirds were smokers and over half of the women had experienced domestic violence in the previous year.

Generally, the community midwives approached the women at the Friday clinic, gave them the information sheet and asked them to think about it. At the next visit to the clinic, the subject was again raised and the women were asked if I could make contact. Those who agreed, and there were very few refusals, were contacted by me by letter, telephone call or visit. Telephones were unreliable, as often the numbers changed or were disconnected between agreeing to the meeting and the date set. Often, I was able to contact women via their mothers; they had telephones and met with their daughters every day. Initial meetings were often at the grandmother's house and grandmothers joined in the discussion. There were many abortive meetings; the women either forgot the arrangement or went out. Mornings were the best times; afternoons were interrupted by the school collection time and evenings totally unacceptable. I had very little control over the sample; I did not use the doctor's lists or invade their privacy by contacting them directly. I only used the telephone if the women had previously agreed with the community midwife to give me the number. There were some elements of a snowball sample technique: some women would tell their friends or just invite themselves along for the chat. I was also invited to the local school summer show. At this meeting, I was able to meet other women who were pregnant or who attended other clinics in the same surgery. I found that 'hanging about' outside the playground at 3.30 in the afternoon opened many more opportunities to collect data and clarify points in the fieldwork. The sample thus had many different starting points.

METHODS, THE WAYS OF GATHERING THE DATA: INTERVIEWS, CONVERSATIONS, CHATS, OBSERVATIONS AND FIELD NOTES

The fieldwork was carried out in 1998-99. A total of 55 in-depth interviews were carried out with 25 white women living in Middleton. These interviews were tape-recorded and transcribed. There was also a series of more informal conversations. Some chats were in groups – again not formal focus groups, but informal meetings and conversations. Most women (some moved away or did not want to bother) were interviewed three times: once during pregnancy, once around the time of the birth, after they had come home from hospital or had recovered from the birth at home, and once some five or six weeks later. Some interviews lasted an hour and a half; other chats or visits lasted only 20 minutes or even less. Whenever possible informal conversations were tape-recorded and transcribed; otherwise I relied on my notebook and memory. The format of the questions varied and the style was open-ended and improvisational. The interviews were conducted in the women's own homes, with others present and the television always on in the background. There were often other children in the room and the grandmother or other friends. I followed up personal introductions, met friends and neighbours, and collected both 'public' and 'private' accounts of women's lives. On one occasion, an interview was conducted whilst a local authority gas fitter repaired the fire, but generally men, related or not, were absent. They would know that I was calling and would quickly get up and leave the room when I arrived. The ages of the women ranged from 15 to 38 years.

The questions were not rigorously pre-planned, or used as part of a questionnaire, but were used to explore feelings, beliefs and values. It was important to respond to each woman as an individual with individual experiences and beliefs. Different women required different questions; I did not try to control or standardise the nature of the interview. Questions were also used to clarify and confirm emerging theories and to explore other issues as they developed. I also kept a detailed fieldwork diary and field notes. I used the basic methodology of the interpretative sociologies: personal observation with varying degrees of participation. Like Jocelyn Cornwall, (1984), I was much more than a recording instrument; the very nature of the relationships I established with the women influenced the content of the interviews. The field notes were completed as soon as possible after any contact in the field. The notes included key aspects of conversations and notes about the environment. Field notes were the record of the participant and non-participant observation that formed a crucial part of the data-collection process. Observation adds breadth to the research and often provided answers to questions that arose from the interviews. The purpose of the observation was to observe the participants in as natural a setting as possible and to describe the settings. My activities are best described as participant-as-observer. I was in and part of the setting, in the GP surgery, in the shops outside the school, at the benefits office etc. I felt that there was little risk of the women behaving differently when I was present; over the weeks and months I observed that their behaviour varied little whoever was present.

I used a hand-held Dictaphone to record key points, reminders and mental notes etc. and wrote up the observations as soon as possible and always the same day. I found it was helpful if I avoided discussing my observations with anyone before I had written them up. Initially I used the guide offered by Lofland and Lofland (1995), and aimed to collect the richest possible data. I recorded what I saw, what I heard, what I smelled, and what I felt and thought during the fieldwork stages. Spradley's (1979, 1980) list of space, actors, activity, objects, acts, events, time, goal and feelings was a useful initial follow-up check. I avoided wherever possible the truncated field note, encouraging myself constantly to record faithfully my observations. The field notes became a wealth of evidence and a series of clues that assisted the analysis.

My checklists were quickly discarded as my observation and interview techniques improved; I allowed the women themselves to lead the interview. I asked less and listened more. As I transcribed the interviews and started the process of analysis I became increasingly impressed with my ability to say very little. The field notes were divided into analytical and substantive notes, written on either side of an A4 notebook, and using different coloured pens. All field notes were typed up and annotated, and represented a running commentary and description of the events. I drew maps and layouts of women's homes, and the health and community centre. Wolcott (1992) describes these research strategies as experiencing (participant observation), enquiring (interviewing) and examining (studying documents). The aim was to collect data that are rich in detail, and provide the so-called 'rich descriptions' that make a sound ethnography.

Throughout the fieldwork stage of this study, I kept a fieldwork diary. I used three headings as a template for my reflections. *Events* were brief summaries of what had happened; the diary complemented my field notes and was useful for checking out the data. *Reactions* was the next heading: I used this mainly to explore my feelings about the day in the field, how I felt about the environment in which I was collecting data, my thoughts about the women I had met and what their stories had taught me. The final heading was *Relevance*. In this section of my diary, I worked on the process of analysis and began to try to understand what it might all mean.

THE ONGOING PROCESS OF ANALYSIS

The analysis of ethnographic data is not a simple one-off activity; it continues throughout the fieldwork stage, the analysis stage and the writing-up stage. Analysis depended on immersion and complete familiarity with the data. There was a need to revisit some women to clarify areas that, prior to another stage of analysis, had seemed clear. The thinking was an almost continuous process, and not one that happened only during an 'analysis stage'.

I initially used the method suggested by Miles and Huberman (1994), utilising multiple copies of all the data. The first step was to affix codes to the field notes, using a highlighter pen and note flags. Comments relating to the data were written in the margin and initial analytical categories were indicated using a coloured pen. The next stage was to sort and sift the material to identify similarities, relationships between various aspects, patterns, emerging themes and common sequences. I used two large sheets of hardboard, a marker pen and numerous sheets of pink paper to sort out this stage. The next stage was to isolate patterns, processes and commonalities in order to move towards elaborating small sets of generalisations that cover consistencies. The final stage was where possible to link these generalisations with an existing body of literature or a formalised theory. Morse and Field (1996) identify the process of analysis as comprehending, synthesising or decontextualising, theorising and recontextualising. The processes occur both sequentially and randomly. All the processes involve long periods of becoming extraordinarily familiar with the data and thinking about the data. As I read and reread the interview data, played and replayed the tapes and retyped my field notes I thought, tried to understand and make sense of the data. The synthesising stage was reached when I felt that I had 'got a feel for the data' and had some feelings about the key areas of the study. I used content analysis to analyse for categories, constructs and domains. I began with thick descriptions and moved on to tabulation, even some descriptive statistics (of the sample); I created classification systems (types of violence, reasons for wanting children etc.), broad categories and subsets of categories. Some categories were abandoned as being too specialised; others were blended together as overlap between the themes became obvious. The main categories eventually became the empirical chapters of the book. The process was complex, demanding, interpretative and reflexive. It did not always follow the neat recipe that Miles and Huberman (1994) describe. I used boxes to store coded data related to the key themes and categories. I also used the simple filing system in Microsoft Word, the word-processing package. I created files named after the key themes, and another called 'other', and transferred marked text from the field notes and interview data to new files. Always I produced hard copies, with sections cut and pasted onto new sheets. I used highlighter pens, notes and different fonts to connect the work.

I considered both *Ethnograph* and *Nud.ist* (Non-Numerical Unstructured Data Indexing, Searching and Theorising) but I found mastering the package detracted from the analysis of the data. I needed to handle the data in its hard copy, physical form in order to deal with the narratives, stories and the emerging and recurring themes. Durkin (1997) argues that QDAs (qualitative data analysis programs) neither promise nor threaten to think; they cannot theorise, nor do they create complex data codes, but they can improve our relationship with the data. This relationship can be circumvented by information technology; I found that the features of a word-processing package supplemented the scissors, glue and highlighter pens. The data collection was organised, systematic and all the data collected are available for scrutiny.

I had initially considered using life histories as a source of data, but the practical difficulties of sitting around long enough to hear the stories proved too great for the women concerned. Some women gave overviews of their childhood and backgrounds, but few could spare the time to explore the past in the detail I required. Many women used the phrase: 'that was then, this is now'. They made it clear that they had no time for thoughtful reflection on the past, or to tell stories of 'what might have been'. There was no need to access medical records; the women told me what they wanted to and, I believe, nothing else. The ethics committee's concerns about confidentiality of medical records became irrelevant. Women willingly showed me their benefit books, their supermarket receipts and credit documentation. They often sought advice on official forms, contracts and letters.

Holstein and Gubrium (1998) state that 'writing up findings from interview data is itself an analytically active enterprise. Rather than adhering to the ideal of letting the data speak for themselves, the active analyst empirically documents the meaning making process'. I avoided the process of summarising and organising the women's words but endeavoured to 'deconstruct participants' talk' to show both the 'hows' and 'whys' of the narratives (Holstein and Gubrium 1998:127). I was also very conscious that as I transcribed the interviews I was punctuating women's accounts. I made the decisions on where to place full stops and commas. I tried always to be true to the women's voices, but my task was interpretative. It was inevitable that sometimes my punctuation would in some minor way change the sense of what I was hearing. Pauses, as indicated by full stops and commas, do not necessarily mean thoughtful reflection, but simply taking a breath. Sometimes women's thoughts came tumbling out without a pause and I was aware that sometimes I added a structure that did not really exist.

Theorising the data was akin to a sorting process; it involved the selection and fitting of the data to the emerging themes. Theorising was the process of constructing alternative explanations and matching such explanations to the data. An example of this was the process of translating women's dramatic accounts of their experience of domestic violence to devising an explanation as to why they remained in abusive relationships and how they sought to avoid life-threatening injuries. Theorising is speculation and best-guessing and provides a means of presenting facts in a useful and pragmatic way. Throughout there was an attempt to link the findings to established theory and to develop theory that could be applied to other women in other settings.

In a small-scale study such as this, the aim was not to produce theory that could be generalised or recontextualised to a different setting. However, the research did seek to increase understanding of the lives of these childbearing women in poverty.

Becoming part of the scene, an insider on the outside, was particularly important. My slightly Welsh accent, sentence construction and vocabulary were obvious barriers. I quickly learned that 'quiche' was not part of the everyday diet in Walsall, and that the question 'Does he knock you about a bit?' was more effective than 'Do you have any direct experience of domestic violence?' I openly explained I was a midwife, but I did not go into details about my academic post or publishing record. I answered questions about my family, my children, and why I came to be living in the Black Country as honestly as possible. I chose to wear informal clothes; leggings and T-shirt with trainers was my usual style of dress. I carried a canvas bag with my notebook, tape recorder, batteries and pens. I once made the mistake of carrying this kit in a Harrods shopping bag. The comments were direct and clear: 'Blimey, that's a bit of a posh bag, innit? Isn't that where Lady Di did her shopping?'

The information sheet explained that the research aimed to improve the midwifery care for women who 'found it hard to make ends meet'; whilst this was not the direct purpose of the research, it is likely that my findings will influence the development of midwifery policy and aspects of care.

Sometimes I found being 'in the field' was traumatic and demanding. I found the smell in some houses overpowering, and I was often irritated by the noise and distractions of children. I have a fear and distaste of large dogs, and other more exotic pets, and this made some aspects of the fieldwork uncomfortable and difficult. I sometimes wanted to shorten an interview knowing that describing and writing up field notes would take yet another day. In many ways, being an outsider on the inside was uncomfortable and demanding. I was often laughed at for not understanding the local vernacular, and asked why I did not do real midwifery any more. I was often frightened by the neighbourhood, and sometimes wondered if the bus would arrive in time to take me away from the site. I gave up using my stylish car for visiting the area at a very early stage in the fieldwork. My wheels had been stolen, and were returned after I had left a pleading note on the windscreen claiming poverty and the fact I was a midwife and engaged in important research about pregnant women. The wheels were returned with a note indicating that the wheels needed balancing to avoid uneven wear. I often wanted to withdraw from the field, but as the study progressed, I adjusted to the environment and to the women themselves. I generally resisted the temptation to help with material possessions, but often took outgrown clothes and toys to some homes. I freely gave midwifery and mothering advice whenever it was sought.

DOING INTERVIEWS

Like Ann Oakley (1995), I found interviewing women was a contradiction in terms. My experiences with women bore very little relationship to the ceremonial order of an organised interview as described in the standard methods texts. Visitors, children, the television, babies crying, hiccups and labour pains interrupted informal conversations. Although I was with the women, being with them to investigate their lives, I felt that my presence did little to interrupt the normal course of events. The traditional warm-up questions, courtesies and polite conversation seemed strangely out of place. One woman anticipated my explanation by saying, 'You have come to find out about what we think for a change, that's okay, I will tell you.' Denzin (1970) describes the need for a balance to be struck between warmth and detachment, friendly but not too friendly, kind but not too kind. This recipe-book approach bears little resemblance to the shambles that formed the backdrop to many encounters. Many women chose the interview to ask me all sorts of questions; the questions ranged from treatment of their grandfather's earwax, to their mother's decision to have a hysterectomy, to the next-door neighbour's experience of a medical termination of pregnancy. In addition, there were numerous questions that related to pregnancy, labour and childbirth. Subsequently, at the local supermarket, some of the women I have worked with have greeted me warmly and proudly shared details of their child's development.

Miller and Glassner (1998), in Silverman (1998:99), state in-depth interviewing can be used to find out about the social world. They reject the arguments put up by radical social constructionists, which suggest that there is no knowledge that can be obtained from an interview about a reality that is 'out there' in the social world. They reject the argument that the interview is obviously and exclusively an interaction between the interviewer and the subject, in which both participants construct narrative versions of the social world, and that narratives are context-specific, invented to fit the demands of the interview and representative only of that context and nothing more. They argue that there is such a thing as truth, and that it can be uncovered using interview techniques. The interviews in this study were carried out simply to generate data that would give an authentic insight into people's experiences and their understanding of the meanings of these experiences (Silverman 1993:91). The aim was always to share the women's subjective view of their experiences, describe them in depth and detail, and in so doing represent those views and feelings as honestly as possible. Arguments that describe the language of interviewing as fracturing the story seem to have very little relevance to my experience. The women in this study were bold individuals who took control of the interview. They had their story to tell and would not be interrupted by my sometimes irrelevant questions. As I became more experienced in the process, my interruptions became fewer; the transcripts are of the women's voices. The researcher's voice was rarely heard and the risk of 'fracturing the stories' was minimal. I believe that the women trusted me, perhaps because I was a midwife, perhaps because I was helpful and came across as being on their side. I had often taken the time to share aspects of my own childhood and my experiences of poverty. This helped to build the rapport and make the encounter less artificial. It took time to build this trust, and the first interviews were sometimes stark and uncomfortable, but the follow-up interviews were free-flowing, energetic and rich in data. Initially, women would check out my background; they were suspicious of the social services, the social worker, the health visitor and the benefit office. They were cautious and defensive at first, but gradually 'sussed out' my interests and concerns. They would often ask me my views on a topic, for example abortion, before they would share their views. Frequently, they would preface their comments by addressing their friend and saying, 'She thinks this too.' The support of the friend was important, especially where a view might be considered contentious. An example might be the frequent discussions on the way the local police force handled drug crime. They commonly complained that the police 'fussed on about car tax discs and television licences' but ignored the open trade in illegal substances on the streets.

Miller and Glassner (1998) challenge Silverman's concerns in respect of 'open-ended interviews' and the need to justify departing from naturally occurring data. His concerns about romantic notions that equate experience with authenticity do not worry Miller and Glassner; they argue that researchers can call upon interviewees' experiences to produce authentic accounts of social worlds. They argue that what matters is an understanding of how stories are produced, the type of stories they are and how they can be used in theorising about social life.

Creative interviewing is a term coined by Holstein and Gubrium (1998) in Silverman (1998). Drawing on the work of Douglas (1985), these authors argue that standard recommendations for conducting research interviews are shallow and ignore the need for a methodology for deep disclosure. The women in this study were, as Douglas describes, 'well guarded vessels of feelings' (1985:51). It was clear that they would not disclose their feelings with men around and not to me until they had the measure of me and my own beliefs and values. I think it probably helped that I was female, overweight and had been brought up as one of five children in a working-class home. There was a clear need to 'get to know the respondents well' and create a climate of mutual disclosure. Sharing thoughts, feelings and experiences was an important part of the process, as was expressing a fascination with the feelings and thoughts of the women and their female relatives. As a female researcher, the process also exposed me to danger; my car was damaged, my purse stolen, and I was attacked with stones by a group of youths. Without the local community midwives, who acted as guides and escorts, the research would not have taken place.

BIAS, OBJECTIVITY, RELIABILITY, VALIDITY AND TRUSTWORTHINESS IN ETHNOGRAPHIC RESEARCH

Bias is closely related to the issue of subjectivity and part of the ongoing debate on objectivity. Feminist researchers have been encouraged to dissolve the distance between themselves and those they research and become reflexive. Such demands are probably unrealistic, and even patronising. The challenge to set aside all those aspects that make the researcher an individual with individual experiences is virtually impossible. According to Scheper-Hughes (1992), the 'cultural self' that every researcher takes into her work is no longer a set of troublesome elements to be eradicated or controlled but rather a set of resources. Sandra Harding (1993) suggests a strategy of 'strong objectivity' that takes the researcher as well as those researched as the focus of critical, causal, scientific explanations. Harding (1991) notes 'strong objectivity requires we investigate the relation between subject and object rather than deny the existence of, or seek unilateral control over this relation' (1991:152). Such a demand goes far beyond any call for reflexivity, and many, e.g. Holland and Ramazanoğlu (1994), argue that it cannot be done. They believe that feminist researchers can only try to explain the grounds on which selective interpretation has been made; they can also make as explicit as possible the processes of decision making that led to the decisions and interpretations.

In 1986, Sandelowski argued that the term *rigour* along with trustworthiness and authenticity are preferable to reliability and validity in qualitative research. However, Anssi Perakyla believes that reliability and validity are important because the objectivity of social science itself is at stake. As more policy decisions are based on qualitative research, objectivity involves ensuring accuracy and inclusiveness of recordings as well as efforts to test out the truthfulness of analytical claims (Perakyla 1998:216). This assumes that achieving objectivity is possible and the truth is accessible, just waiting to be uncovered. It assumes there is a single underlying explanation; it only requires uncovering. The view taken in this research is that there can be no 'truth', only further steps along the way of understanding.

LeCompte and Goetz (1982) identify critical areas where external reliability could be affected: the status or position of the researcher, the informant choices, the social context in which the data are gathered, the definitions of the constructs and their relationships, and the methods of data gathering and analysis. Kirk and Miller (1986), on the other hand, point out that in conducting and assessing qualitative research, the primary emphasis has usually been laid on validity rather than reliability. They define reliability as 'the degree to which the finding is independent of accidental circumstances of the research' (1986:20). In ethnographic research, assessing the reliability of the research results entails whether or not (or under what conditions) the ethnographer would expect to obtain the same finding if he or she tried again in the same way. Independent repetition is the ideal way of assessing reliability, but unrealistic in an ethnographic study.

Validity of research concerns the interpretation of observations and whether or not the researcher is calling what is measured by the right name. Threats to external validity are those effects that obstruct or reduce a study's comparability. Morse and Field (1996) argue that synthesising the results of studies that examine the same phenomena but in different contexts and then comparing and contrasting the results enhances external validity. Lincoln and Guba (1985) suggest the crucial test for ethnographic accounts is whether the respondents, whose beliefs and behaviour they are describing, recognise the validity of those accounts. Their model addresses four aspects: truth-value, applicability, consistency and neutrality. Truth-value or credibility is important, but must be seen in the context of multiple realities; applicability is used to determine whether the findings can be applied to other settings; consistency is discovered if the study is replicated, assuming that both the actors and the environment remain unchanged; neutrality is the freedom of bias in the research, established by the researchers' willingness to identify their own biases through reflexivity and through consultation with other researchers and supervisors. According to Bloor (1978:548-9) the aim in seeking credibility is to 'establish a correspondence between the sociologists and the member's social world by exploring the extent to which members recognise, give assent to, the judgements of the sociologist' (cited in Hammersley and Atkinson 1995).

Sandelowski (1993) has moved away from her initial focus on rigour. In her later paper she believes there is an uncompromising harshness and rigidity in the term rigour that is too far from the 'artfulness, versatility and sensitivity to meaning and context that mark qualitative works of distinction' (cited in Morse and Field 1996). To subject studies to repetition can be useless as both the informants and the context of the study will inevitably have changed.

Feeding back the findings to the respondents can assess validity. In this research, this was difficult but not impossible to achieve. I offered all women a copy of the transcribed interview, and a few said they would look at it; most asked me to summarise what I saw as the key issues. I did this for each interview and for each woman. I showed them all a one-page summary of the key themes and encouraged them to comment. I took the time to explore my interpretation of the accounts with the respondents. I encouraged discussion and checked out my assumptions. Finally I offered to give them a summary of the research and a note of what I would be sharing with other midwives and researchers. Others must judge issues of trustworthiness.

Finally, Richardson (1993) offers an alternative and more hopeful view on the subject of validity in qualitative research. She says:

'I challenge different kinds of validity and call for different kinds of science practices. The science practice I model is a feminist-post-modern one. It blurs genres, probes lived experiences, enacts science, creates a female imagery, breaks down dualisms, inscribes female labour and emotional responses as valid, deconstructs the myth of an emotion-free social science and makes space for partiality, self reflexivity, tension and difference' (1993:695).

This reflects my beliefs and experience of ethnographic research in Middleton. It was always my intention to respect the women I worked with, to appreciate their contribution and willingness to help and to respect their experiences. I aim to present their accounts with sensitivity and a reflexive eye.

LEAVING THE FIELD

I experienced mixed feelings at the end of the fieldwork stage of the research. In many ways I did not leave as I continued to live and shop in the area. The process of withdrawal was gradual; I continued to visit the Friday clinic for some months after the fieldwork, just to talk to the women, to see who had had their baby and answer any questions. I put up a notice in the clinic to thank all the women and let the women know that I had completed the work. I also offered to meet anyone who still wanted to see me. I also left a brief summary of the study and my telephone number at home and work.

SUMMARY

This chapter has described the methodology used in this research and, through a thread running through the chapter, I have debated the various views and debates in the related literature. I have used the framework to guide my progress through the process and as a tool for analysis of the findings. I have described the process of seeking approval in a research world dominated by positivist scientists and medical control. I have described the realities of researching a disadvantaged group and have explained how I have sought to value and respect the women who contributed to the study.

Olesen in Olesen and Clarke (1999) states:

'It is important to recognise that knowledge production is continually dynamic – new frames open which give way to others which in turn open again and again. Moreover, knowledges are only partial. Some may find these views discomfiting and see them as a slippery slope of ceaseless constructions with no sure footing for action of whatever sort. It is not that there is no platform for action, reform, transformation or emancipation but the platforms are transitory. If one's work is overturned or altered by another researcher with a different, more effective approach, then one should rejoice and move on.

What is important for concerned feminists is that new topics, issues for concern and matters for feminist inquiry are continually produced and given attention to yield more nuanced understandings on critical issues' (1999:356).

In the chapters that follow, I will explore some new topics; I will examine the changing nature of the relationship between childbearing women and the men in their lives and an understanding of the tactics some women adopt as they remain in abusive relationships. In the next chapter, I consider some issues around motherhood and explore the ways in which some of the women in this study viewed motherhood as part of a life struggling to cope with the daily grind of poverty.

4

Exploring motherhood: responsibility and respectability in Middleton

INTRODUCTION

In this chapter, I explore what I found to be the key recurring themes of responsibility and respectability; I first set the scene and describe some aspects of the environment where the study takes place. I explore the meanings of motherhood and consider how middle-class discourses are used to construct the social codes for other classes. I draw on the work of Kaplan (1992), who charts the contesting and contradictory discourses of motherhood in North American literature and culture, and the work of Sharon Hays (1996) who explores how working mothers in the 1990s face the challenge of being both nurturing and unselfish at home as mothers, whilst being competitive and ambitious at work. The ideology of 'intensive mothering' exacerbates the tensions that face working mothers. I discuss the work of Ann Phoenix (1991) to illustrate that although teenage motherhood is deeply ingrained in the public consciousness as a social problem, the main problem of young and single mothers is poverty. I then present some findings from this research to explore women's feelings about motherhood and to demonstrate their strong sense of responsibility. Putting children first was as important to these women as it was to the working mothers in Hay's study who were caught up in 'intensive mothering'. The meaning of motherhood and the classed meanings, i.e. women as socially excluded, are considered in the context of the milieu in which they live and bring up their children. The costs of striving to be respectable and being responsible whilst living in poverty are immense. I then draw on the work of McMahon (1995) to illustrate how the notion of choice is inadequate in understanding motherhood. Drawing on data from interviews and observation I then explore some of the women's motivations to motherhood. Responsibility was seen as a key theme, as was motherhood as a route to respectability. Having children was also seen as a route to happiness, to negate the effects of poverty and as a form of compensation for the hardship of material deprivation. In the final section, I explore how women in this study balanced the needs of their children with the demands of a life dominated by poverty and how being a 'good mother' brought some sense of satisfaction, respectability, personal worth and self-esteem.

(A summary of the details of the sample of women who contributed to the study is included in 'Introducing the Women'. Each woman was allocated a number and details of name, age, marital status, previous pregnancies etc. have been recorded. All the names have been changed to preserve anonymity.)

LEARNING MORE ABOUT MIDDLETON

In ethnographic research, the analysis of data begins almost at the start of the process. Analysis is part of the pre-fieldwork thinking, part of the collecting of field notes and memos and part of the writing-up. As I became more deeply involved in the culture of Middleton I knew, at times, that I was in danger of losing my outsider view and even 'going native'. It was important to retreat to my middle-class home and write in detail about the world of childbearing women living in poverty. At first I wrote in detail about anything that struck me as different – different from my own life style or different from my understanding or experience. I generated vast quantities of field notes, reflections and memos and started to write more about the lives, beliefs and values of the women of the study who were living in Middleton. I also studied aspects of their culture and the environment in which they lived. The culture is 'the way we do things around here' or the beliefs, customs, conventions, the language or way of life of the group. Hammersley and Atkinson (1995) describe the sense of alienation and 'strangeness' experienced by field workers studying the strange and exotic. Bowen (1954), in Hammersley and Atkinson (1995), describes the feelings of incompetence and the pain in coming to terms with the estrangement of researching a new social setting. I recognise and understand the strength of 'culture shock'. In the setting I was an 'acceptable incompetent' – acceptable because I was a midwife, but also because the women were tolerant of my intrusion and faintly amused at my attempts to uncover what was for them a normal part of everyday life. I was aware that sometimes I was shocked by what I saw and heard, but throughout the study, I aimed to be sensitive, thoughtful and reflexive. I recognised and valued my subjectivity and I consciously tried to avoid being judgemental.

Middleton is a white-dominated, deprived and run-down area with an unemployment rate of 20 per cent (in some parts of Middleton the rate is 26 per cent). It is an area where 37.7 per cent of the population describe their health as bad or very bad and where the majority of homes, owned by the local authority, are in need of repair. The houses were three- and four-bedroom semi-detached or terraces. There were also some small blocks of maisonettes each containing four or six flats built no more than two storeys high. Most of the women and their families were registered with one GP, a single-handed practice with a practice nurse, a practice manager and a team of community midwives. They all used the same local benefits office, local post office, the local 'chippy', the 'bookie' and most of the children attended the same junior and senior schools. All the women in the study complained at the same neighbourhood office. They complained about the rent, the need for repairs and their lack of progress up the waiting list for rehousing, the noisy neighbours and the drug abuse that was going on outside their front doors. They all shopped at the local shop, 'The Happy Shopper', for occasional needs like a pint of milk. It was this local shop that took milk tokens, and most women used the shop to exchange the tokens. Most complained that the owner was dishonest in calculating the difference between litres and pints but they continued to use the shop for convenience. They all bought their lottery tickets in the same newsagent, usually between £5 and £8 worth per week. The lottery could be seen as a measure of desperateness as the amount spent on tickets seemed to reflect the urgency for more money. One woman who was expecting the bailiffs to call the following Monday spent £11 on lottery tickets as a last resort. She did not win and is probably unlikely to attend a performance at the newly refurbished, lottery-funded Royal Opera House, or go to see a ballet. This redistribution of wealth from the poor to the rich was brought into sharp focus on the Middleton estate.

In the sense of sharing facilities and geographical location, the women who lived in Middleton could be described as a community. But shared actions do not necessarily mean that a group of people share experiences or a common identity, for many of the residents of this Middleton housing estate saw themselves as temporary residents. In the group of women I studied, not one had lived in the area for more than two years. All expected or aspired to move on to a better area as soon as they could. Life in Middleton is loosely connected; some women expressed no sense of companionship with other women on the estate, and individually they all expressed the need to move on. Others shared their lives with other women. Outside the primary school, women would talk to their mothers and sometimes they would exchange a word with their neighbour. In this ethnography, men were generally absent; it was the women who quietly got on with the business of bringing up children as well as creating and building homes.

Hilary Graham (1987b), in her work on poverty and lone mothers, describes how women controlled their income and expenditure in such a way as to gain control over their lives. In this study, it was the women who appeared to feel the sharp pain of living in such a poor environment and who coped daily with the drudgery of poverty. Some of the women I worked with had no means of escape; they could not leave the area, go to the pub or see their 'mates' without their children. They were responsible for their children and for building their home in bleak circumstances. One woman told me that more than anything she wanted a shed; she wanted a small private place that was hers and only hers where she could escape for some peace and quiet.

Middleton is a much run-down area. More than 1 in 15 of the entire working population had been unemployed for over a year (Walsall Public Health Report 1996). The mortality rate of those under 65 is 65 per cent higher than the average for England and Wales. The houses were in a poor state of repair with many boarded up with metal sheets covering the windows. The gardens were generally overgrown and unkempt and filled with discarded bicycles, furniture, beds, bricks, plaster, rusty iron, discarded refrigerators, washing machines and general household refuse. There were a number of burnt-out and abandoned cars and cars dismantled and being repaired. There were frequently the signs of a bonfire smouldering and the smell of burnt tyres. The streets were covered in litter and the road signs rendered illegible by graffiti. More than one fifth of the houses are considered by the council to be unfit for human habitation. In some houses, there was a car in the drive, neat curtains and freshly painted woodwork. In one house that was owned by a retired couple, there was a caravan. The area was frightening; on the street corners were groups of young men. I always felt afraid and uncomfortable.

One distinctive feature of the area was the physical appearance of the inhabitants; many were overweight. Walsall has a greater number of overweight people than any other area in the UK; the local and national media refer to the inhabitants as 'Walsall Wobblies'. To me the inhabitants looked pale-faced and strained; their children seemed to my maternal and professional eyes somewhat pale and tired. I felt that the women were coping with a difficult life but these observations merely reflect my own subjectivity and the contrast that existed between their lives and mine. In one part of the estate the houses were built around a patch of grass; there were no trees but the local 'tat' man would park his van on the patch of grass and lay out his wares for sale. The 'tat' man bought clothing and household goods from jumble sales, the local tip and charity shops; these goods were sorted and sold at very low prices from his van. Baby clothes were very popular: a 'babygro' would be five pence, a bib two pence and a vest two pence. The environment was hostile and challenging and it was in this environment that they sought to bring up their children, take control of their lives and be seen as respectable women and mothers. I found the environment challenging and the research work difficult. Although the women were friendly and, as the study progressed, helpful and kind, it was a hostile environment and I was an outsider intruding into their lives.

EXPLORING THE MEANING OF MOTHERHOOD: DISCOURSES OF MOTHERHOOD AT HOME AND ABROAD

Motherhood was central to the lives of the women. This study would not and could not discover a universal truth about poverty nor about motherhood but it can add to our understanding of how these complex concepts act together. The discourses on motherhood and mothering are worthy of consideration.

MOTHERHOOD IN AMERICA

Kaplan (1992) has analysed aspects of popular culture and drama and discusses the contesting and contradictory discourses of the mother in America. She analysed the ways in which mothers have been represented in three related spheres: the historical, charting representations in literature and films from 1830 to postmodernist days; the psychoanalytical; and how the mother is figured in literary and film texts. She charts the discourses of the mother through cultural perspectives. She argues that the period from 1970 to 1990 was a period of intense transition; she believes that the overall change was closely linked to childbirth and child care. It became clear that, unlike the past when women's biological and reproductive roles were unquestioned, childbirth and childrearing were no longer being viewed as an automatic, natural part of woman's life cycle. She has shown the emergence, in representations, of the angel/witch mother dichotomy and how representations in different decades played on the unconscious fears of the mother. Mothers had a clear role and function; they should bear and nurture children for the good of society, and indeed without them the social order itself was under threat. Kaplan argues that the anxiety emerges as women can now decide whether or not to mother and what sort of context mothering wants or needs. As childbearing is no longer automatic, the range of options open to women creates anxiety. She gives particular attention to the changing nature of advertisements for Mother's Day gifts and notes that it is the white middle-class discourses which are used to register the dominant social codes that in turn implicate or construct the social codes for other classes and social groups. In her survey of Mother's Day advertisements she found that initially household goods were suggested as gifts; this changed to 'sexy' nightgowns, dresses and perfume. She argues that by 1986 women had won the right to be both mother and 'sexy'. By 1988 babies were included in advertisements; later, consumer goods such as cameras, camcorders and videos were added. Her belief is that white middle-class norms such as the place of women, glamour, sex and power are reflected in advertisements. These advertisements offer images of women as mothers, which change to reflect the latest view, the latest discourses on the place and role of women. The women portrayed in these and other advertisements are usually white and middle class. It is these women who set the standards for others to follow and thus define the norm. She discusses the discourses of the 'absent mother' and the 'nurturing father' and the tensions that surround the working mother and explores the ways in which mothers are still blamed far more than fathers for what goes wrong with children. She analyses how the cultural codes continue to promote the belief that 'good' mothers cannot be good workers.

DISCOURSES ON MOTHERHOOD AND CHILD CARE: A 'GOOD' MOTHER

The discourses about child care continue to raise concerns about the effects of day care on the psychic health of the child and the concerns that the growing numbers of working women threaten family values or even the institution of the family itself. In discourses about 'abusive and neglectful' mothers, mothers are blamed, as individuals, rather than blame being placed on inadequate social structures and government priorities that have steered funds in other directions.

Kaplan (1992) argues that there are predominant representations about, and addressed to, the poor that usually speak from an implicit, judgemental, middle-class position. The women in this study are blamed and patronised by health professionals who hold them responsible personally for their own poor health and that of their children. If they work they are neglectful; if they stay at home they are 'benefit scroungers'; if they choose childlessness they risk being called selfish. There is, it appears, a right time to be a mother, and a 'right' social class that should be encouraged to have children and bring them up. The right time is when a child can be afforded and the woman supported by a man, a luxury only achieved by the middle classes.

In the 1990s, discourses about lesbian mothers revealed outmoded assumptions about the effects of a lesbian household on children and implied difficulties for the children involved. Kaplan goes on to assert that in the late twentieth century, the images, the literature and the discourses led to contrary images of women fulfilling themselves through childbearing. Motherhood was no longer a duty but fulfilling. Kaplan has demonstrated that what it means to be a mother and what is expected of women in their roles as mothers changes significantly over time. She argues that modern reproductive technologies have created dramatic changes in the representation of the mother figure. The message to women is both confusing and contradictory. The dominant discourses are complex, but they are formulated with white, middle-class women as the focus and they are powerful in instructing women from other social classes and ethnic groups about what they should do and how they should live their lives.

INTENSIVE MOTHERING

Intensive mothering is a logically cohesive combination of beliefs, which include being a dedicated mother. It means spending the 'correct' amount of time with the child and carefully choosing the correct 'alternate mothers' in day care. It means breast-feeding her child, reading to the child, and taking the child to ballet class and swimming. It means that the mother is completely responsible for the child's behaviour and is ready to 'kill and die' for her child. It means that discipline is carefully controlled and discussed and that her love is powerful, spilling over into her paid working life. As a mother, she is responsible for the costs of child care, education, vacations, the enhancement of family life and the requirements of socially appropriate childrearing.

In the example of Rachel, used by Hays (1996), Rachel has two different worlds: the world of home where her nurturing side is used and the world of work which is 'public, cold and uncaring'. Hays argues that 'intensive mothering' is a powerful, historically constructed, contemporary ideology that is both contradictory and oppressive. She focuses on middle-class women in America who, as mothers with young children, work in often well-paid positions. She argues that whilst it is accepted that women will contribute to the labour market many are still unsure whether they approve of this state of affairs. She believes that the ideology of intensive mothering is a gendered model that advises mothers to expend an enormous amount of time, energy and money in raising their children. She believes that in a society where the logic of self-interested gain seems to guide the behaviour in so many spheres of life, one might wonder why a logic of unselfish nurturing guides the behaviour of mothers. Hays analysed the history of ideas about childrearing and looked at the logic underpinning appropriate mothering and social contexts. She conducted a textual analysis of contemporary childrearing manuals to find the underlying themes and finally she talked to mothers about their childrearing practices. It is in these accounts that the diversity amongst mothers becomes evident. There are differences amongst individual women and differences that follow social class backgrounds. There were similarities as well as differences as the concept of 'appropriate childrearing' was clarified. She considers how paid working mothers and 'stay at home' mothers made sense of their respective positions but demonstrates that the differences between the two groups were complex, although both groups shared a deep commitment to the ideology of intensive childrearing. She argues that:

'The ideology of intensive mothering is promoted and respected because it holds a fragile but nonetheless powerful cultural position as the last best defence against what many people see as the impoverished social ties, communal obligations, and unremunerated commitment' (Hays 1996:xiii).

Hays explores how every mother's ideas about mothering are shaped by a complex map of her class position, race, heritage, religious background, political beliefs, sexual preferences, physical abilities or disabilities, citizenship status, participation in various subcultures, place of residence, work-place environment, formal education, the techniques her parents used to raise her and more (1996:76). For working-class mothers, Hays believes that mothering was one of the more meaningful and socially valued tasks in which they might engage. Both working mothers and 'stay at home' mothers demonstrated an equal commitment to serious mothering. Hays argues that the mass of information and advice on appropriate childrearing, much of it recommending intensive mothering, fundamentally shapes the way mothers think about mothering. I believe that the women living in poverty in this study face similar pressures to be a 'good mother'; some women explained to me how they were anxious to secure the approval of the health and social care professionals as sometimes they believed that approval would result in better care. But these women have to be good mothers whilst coping with poverty, debt, and the effects of poor housing and dismal local facilities. To be a good mother is to be part of an inclusive society. It means taking responsibility and commanding respect and it is a clear route to a superior moral status.

MOTHERHOOD IN MIDDLETON

Faced with these discourses, contradictions and pressures, I wanted to study what motherhood meant to these women themselves. As childbearing women living in poverty, they were well aware of the attitudes of health professionals who questioned their ability and even their right to be mothers (this is explored in chapter eight). They were well aware of the dominating parenting discourses that stress the 'right' time to be a parent. Right is determined according to perceived maturity, readiness and economic stability. As in Ann Phoenix's (1991) study, the right time to have a baby is when the woman is physically mature, supported and financially stable. The women in this study explained how they were aware of these codes and rules but felt that they should and could act independently. I was not able to uncover a universal rule for becoming a mother; what I did discover was that there were many different reasons and motivations for motherhood amongst these women.

It was Maria [19], a 17-year-old single woman, who said:

'I knew everyone would disapprove of me, unless you are old enough, married, he has a good job and you have a home you should not do it, [laughs] you shouldn't do it or have a baby ... well bugger that.'

Initially the women in this study appeared to view motherhood as just another drain on their lives and resources. They complained about the physical strain, always feeling tired, the cost of nappies, 'another mouth to feed', and the interrupted nights. But there was much more to motherhood than the physical effects and as I became more involved with their lives and spent more and more time listening to them I was able to uncover more about their experiences and beliefs about motherhood. For some motherhood was seen as 'natural' or the right thing to do; it was, as they said, what they were born to do but for others it was more complex. Some women talked about motherhood from many perspectives. They developed their views, beliefs and explanations during interviews and between visits; their motivations were complex and varied. I believe there is no simple theory that explains why women living in poverty choose motherhood; most *did* choose motherhood. Their children were not always 'accidents' or irresponsible acts.

Sara Delamont challenges the view that motherhood is 'natural' or the 'right' thing to do at any stage of life. She explores both the contradictions and absurdities of motherhood in this quotation:

'All rational, adult women want to be mothers in wedlock, so all married women want babies, and no unmarried women do. This basic belief leads to a series of correlated ideas, so that the "problem" of the unmarried mother is "solved" if she marries; that married women do not want children are "unnatural" or ill or "selfish"; and socially most crucial, that because women are "driven" to maternity by biological urges, all offspring of married women are "really" wanted' (1980:198).

Thus it appears that all 'natural' women will have a 'natural' maternal instinct that drives them to motherhood. This is unlike men, who are not assumed to have any 'natural' paternal instinct but are driven solely by their biological drives. Images of motherhood as caring, responsible and self-sacrificing are transmitted through the media and mothers are expected to be warm, kind and understanding. Fathers, it seems, can be absent or play a small part in the day-to-day task of childrearing.

For some years, feminists have referred to the 'myth of motherhood'. Whilst motherhood is a natural biological state, it is given a far greater significance and status in society. Motherhood, like other ideological constructs, has taken on the appearance of a natural phenomenon and it is assumed to be the natural state to which all women aspire. Sheila Rowbotham (1974) contests the belief that happiness comes only through motherhood and believes that it should be challenged as a myth that denies women choices and other possibilities. Motherhood, she argues, is both oppressive and fulfilling and must be freely chosen.

TEENAGE MOTHERHOOD

Ann Phoenix in her 1991 study of young mothers addresses the moral panic that surrounds 'teenage motherhood'. She argues that its definition as a social problem is deeply ingrained into the public consciousness yet the evidence in terms of physical consequences does not support the level of concern. The reality is that so-called 'young mothers' are probably at the peak of their childbearing potential; they are physically better equipped to withstand pregnancy than their older women friends. According to Phoenix (1991), the women and their children in her study were mostly doing fine; lack of money was their major problem and in view of their educational and family background that would not have improved if they had delayed motherhood until later. Furstenberg (1992) neatly points out that having children in the teenage years may not cause poverty or disadvantage, but doing so decreases the odds of avoiding either. Published research on young mothers assumes a universal experience of teenage motherhood and suggests universal solutions. Assumptions are linked to the notions of the deserving and undeserving benefit claimants discussed in the Introduction. The moral panic is often linked to the feelings that the social security budget is running wildly out of control paying benefits to feckless, irresponsible *'girls'* who choose the path of motherhood whilst either too young or unsupported by a *'man'*.

In Ann Phoenix's study most of the women in her sample were poorly educated and had experienced high rates of unemployment before they became pregnant. Phoenix (1991) examines how women came to be mothers. Their accounts indicated that they had become pregnant and had chosen to give birth for a variety of reasons. These reasons ranged from having 'planned' their pregnancies to not having considered that they were likely to become pregnant. Young women are often presumed to have become pregnant because they had insufficient knowledge about sex and contraception, yet none of the women interviewed here had become pregnant through ignorance of contraception. All knew the different kinds of contraception that were available. It is clear that the issues are much more complex than having sufficient knowledge. Tracey illustrates this well.

Tracey [12], a 29-year-old mother of five children, described her feelings about motherhood and the views of the 'authorities' who were trying to arrange for her to be sterilised:

'**I am waiting to be sterilised [baby two weeks old]. But I am not going. It's not like being a proper woman is it? You know if you see every month and not be able to catch. The pill is no good, I forget more than I take, and that injection gives me bad headaches. He won't go he hates hospitals. Sterilisation it ain't right, it ain't normal. I love my kids and I'll always want more.**

They always send for me [for the operation], but I don't go. I have no intention of going, but I say I will to get them off my back. I have moved eight times in the past five years, if you keep moving the letters get lost and they give

up nagging you. I won't get sterilised and that's that.

You will never be lonely with kids, at Christmas and you will always be happy. Of course it's a struggle but one more don't make no difference. It's someone to love. It's what I am, I am a mother. Why should hospital tell me when to stop having any more?'

Tracey clearly demonstrates that she has an adequate knowledge of contraceptive methods; for her the decision to have children was far more complex. Being a 'proper woman' or a 'natural' woman is part of the motherhood myth. Tracey believed that her 'natural' state was to be a mother and to continue to be capable of motherhood.

In Phoenix's study (1991), there was no evidence that young women became pregnant in order to get council housing or social security benefits – a position mirrored in this study and reflected in one of the interviews with Emma [25]:

'Anyone who thinks that anyone would go through this just for a flat must be mad. It's not just the cost of the flat is it? You have to buy furniture, heating, electric and all that. The cost of nappies is enough on its own. It's just daft to think that anyone would be mother just to get somewhere to live and some money. Politicians all think we are daft. There is always this feeling that because we live here that we are just not good enough.'

In Phoenix's study all of the women, except one, found child care relatively easy and unproblematic. All reported that they loved their children. Children's needs were reported to be the most important in the hierarchy of the household and several women reported that they went without to ensure that the child's needs were met. This is again mirrored in this study; the women had a very well developed sense of responsibility towards their children. In fact, it could be argued that they were over-responsible. They often went without even during pregnancy. They, like the women in Phoenix's study, loved their children and were determined to provide for them. They accepted the dominant ideologies in western societies, which suggest that childhood should be a commercialised period with educational toys (i.e. computers) and smart (i.e. designer and labelled) clothing should be provided for children. Phoenix explains that poverty made the acceptance of such ideologies oppressive. Women went without themselves and provided what they could.

MOTHERHOOD IN CANADA (AND MIDDLETON)

Martha McMahon (1995) explores the meanings and experiences of motherhood in a group of 59 mothers in Canada. She discusses the ways in which motherhood is a moral transformation of self but describes how this works differently in middle-class and working-class women. Whilst middle-class women see motherhood as confirming their already moral nature, for working-class and poor women it is the route to a superior moral state. She explores the rewards and costs of motherhood and the impact of motherhood on women's identities. She investigated how women's sense of themselves was transformed through the process of becoming mothers. She describes how she inverts the conventional ideas of how mothers produce children and looks instead at how children produce mothers. She argues that motherhood is far more than an expression of female identity but it is the experience of motherhood that produces a gendered sense of self. McMahon argues that there are difficulties in juggling the negative and positive interpretations of motherhood in feminism; it is a paradox that motherhood can be both a women's weakness and strength. She argues that there is no single meaning of motherhood and no unified position. In her work she demonstrates how for some women their sense of identity was deeply implicated in their transition to maternity; it had far more meaning than simply maximising satisfaction. She showed how women followed very different paths to motherhood and developed very different conceptions of themselves as mothers.

In one example in my research, one woman initially explained that her motivation to motherhood was merely to follow her sisters. They had had children, seemed to enjoy it, so she followed suit. In subsequent meetings this explanation was dismissed; as I became more involved with her she explained that being a mother gave her status and authority that she could not find elsewhere. In McMahon's terms, it first appeared that she had been socialised or internalised the norms and values of a culture to provide a blueprint for living. This is an inadequate explanation and does not do justice to the complexity of decisions facing women. Becoming a mother is far more than a conditioned response; in this study, as in McMahon's, women followed quite different routes to motherhood. In McMahon's study of working-class women she found that working-class women were more likely to say 'I have always wanted to be a mother.' Motherhood was taken for granted and the issue was 'when' rather than 'whether'. This was expressed by the women in this research. Sharon [9] said:

'I wanted to be a mother when I was three. I had a doll's pram for Christmas and a doll that wet and cried. I knew then I wanted to be a mum; it's my earliest memory I think. When my Mum had my sister, I was so impressed with what she could do. Being a Mum makes you important.

It's what I have always wanted, I couldn't wait really.'

In McMahon's study, for some women the need to claim the identity of mother was important, as was the positive identity associated with being a mother. Others were particularly attracted to the positive images of motherhood, a view reflected in Joanna's [22] comments:

'I couldn't wait to get pregnant at first. It was like an adventure. I was wrapped up in the planning. I wanted the very best pram, the best cot, and the best Moses basket. I used to drool over the catalogues. I didn't have much money but I worked extra shifts and double time on Sunday to buy all the gear. I remember being really excited about baby vests, booties, and cardigans. I even bought a car seat, we didn't have a car. But it was all exciting. I didn't want anything second hand, especially for the first. Buying stuff was really exciting.'

McMahon found that working-class women were less likely to have been surprised by motherhood than middle-class women were. She explains that motherhood for both classes of women provided them with symbolic resources for the transformation of deeply felt senses of self. For working-class women in McMahon's study, becoming a mother was seen as becoming almost a new person; they felt that they had a moral worth and a position in society. They articulated this sense through language of 'responsibility' and 'settling down'. McMahon summarises her work by saying that motherhood is a more unsettling, complex, important and politically challenging research issue than she had imagined. The notion of choice is hopelessly inadequate for understanding motherhood. In the following examples, it can be seen that becoming a mother was a complex issue. It was never simply a lack of knowledge about contraception or a contraceptive accident. The motivations were complex and linked to so many aspects of their lives. It took some time to be able to talk to women about such complex and intimate issues; in time the women became friends and talked openly about their lives and motherhood. I asked them about being mothers and about their motivations and feelings. Their answers were as varied as the women themselves. This is what they said.

Mel [1]

'I really enjoyed being pregnant the first time. It was just the feeling, the baby growing inside you, it felt good. I did

not plan this one, but all my pregnancies were contraception mess ups. But I still love them. You get a bit of respect being a mother, I got more confident really. You know if anyone has a go at you, as a mother you have a go back. You protect your kids, that makes you feel good.'

Rachel [2]

'I was in a dead end, go nowhere job, sticking handles on saucepans, I hated it, it was going nowhere. I remember thinking I don't want to do this for the rest of my life. I've no qualifications. I met M. It seemed a good idea. We didn't plan it, but I love it all, I love the shopping, the planning, and all that stuff. I have bought a cot, a pram, and all the clothes. It makes me feel good. I shout "I am a mother", no one can take that away.'

Sarah [8]

'I want babies to look after me when I'm old. You've got things to look forward to when you have a child. When it's Christmas, see their faces when they open their presents, birthdays. When you don't have kids you don't have anything to look forward to. It's Christmas, you get enjoyment out of it.'

Maria [19]

'Well it makes me feel good about myself; you have to have kids to feel that. Something to look forward to, if you had no kids there ... is nobody to visit you. You ain't got nothing, have you?'

Joanna [22]

'With kids you have grand children to look forward to, grand kids to buy things for. If I didn't have kids, it was just me there would be nothing. Nothing to live for really.'

Hayley [23]

'After the accident [had a road accident and fracture in the previous year], I thought if I was ill or old there would be nobody to look after me. I love it, I feel like a woman now, not a girl. I have some respect I suppose. I love all the baby things, buying all the things the prams and that.'

Gaynor [18]

'After I had been knocked about and beaten up by F I really wanted someone to love me for me, you know, someone who needed me and would love me, not hurt me. When I split up with F I knew I wanted a baby, it didn't matter about the man, I wanted someone who would love me, be mine and no one else's.'

And Tracey [12]

'It's for love really I never had love I was put into care when I was three years old. It's just to love them and love them back when they love you. I want to be a better parent than my mother was to me I want to achieve more than my mother. I am going to have more and more. As long as they have love, loved fed and clothed ... you can't do more. I try to bring them up right; they never go short of anything. They have loads of toys. I get them what they need ... somehow.'

The themes of responsibility are clear: responsibility for being a parent, for having someone to love. Responsibility led to 'a bit of respect' and to able to 'feel good'. 'I try to bring them up right' reflects the importance of responsibility to the women in this study. They did not consider that there was a right time to become a mother, and they disregarded any suggestion that they might be considered irresponsible in becoming mothers. In fact, motherhood was seen as a route to becoming responsible and with that the ability to command respect.

For these women, it seems that children are about many things: pleasure, status, becoming a woman, respect, self-esteem, love, about having a purpose and meaning in life, having something to be owned exclusively, an insurance against loneliness in later life, a way out of an inadequate job, even a guarantee of a good Christmas. It made women feel good about themselves and made them feel stronger about facing challenges from others. It seems that, for these women, motherhood is a fixed, unalterable structure. All these aspects can be seen as negating the effects of poverty. Children were in some way a compensation for the hardship of material deprivation. They did not feel good about themselves without children. The poverty and material deprivation made their lives hard and uncomfortable.

Becoming a mother was part of the search for pleasure and happiness in a largely intolerable life. Being a mother was seen as part of being a woman, and according to Tracey, to be sterilised made her less than a proper woman. As previously stated, I found no evidence at all of women becoming pregnant to secure accommodation. It is sometimes described as myth, but in this sample motherhood appeared to be woman's inevitable destiny. The fact that happiness came through motherhood illustrates how these women were denied, by poverty or other deprivation, of any other possibilities.

I asked Debbie [15], a 19-year-old single woman and mother of three children, about her life with children and her feelings about motherhood:

'If I could put the clock back I probably would not have children so young. I know I could have gone to college and done a secretarial course or something. I was clever in school, good at English at things. I got pregnant by accident, well a sort of accident. I didn't mind really, I sort of knew it would happen. It seemed exciting; it was getting away from school, from teachers and rules. For once I would be in charge. I would rather have them young ... they grow up with you and then you get a life to yourself. I am really proud of them. It takes all my time and my energy. I get them up, do their breakfast, get them dressed and clean the house. I take pride in the house but every day is the same. Making a loaf last till payday. Going without on Wednesday, always doing without because something comes up, new shoes for the kids, or a bill to pay. I would love to buy some clothes for me in a proper shop, but the kids come first. The kids will look after me when I am old. You have got things to look forward to with kids. It makes me feel good about myself. You have to have kids to feel that. When you get old ... if you have no kids there would be nobody to visit you. You ain't got nothing then.'

MANAGING THE MONEY IN MIDDLETON

The women I spoke to have lives dominated by financial problems; all of them were in debt and all said that they ran out of money at the end of the week. Throughout the interviews, it was obvious that children came first and providing for their children was a major source of their stress and anxiety. They were responsible for their children and although they tried to get the state, the health services and their partners to help, it was clear that they shouldered the burden of responsibility. The women in this study often expressed their responsibilities for their children in terms of their love. Mother love was demonstrated by their commitment to their children and in the energy they invested in the relationship. Skeggs (1997) argues that responsibility, for children, homes and families, provides women with respectability. Not having children or a job and living in your mother's house fails to provide women with an opportunity to have responsibility. Doing 'mothering' well is part of the search for respectability and thus social inclusion in a life where poverty and social class has created social exclusion. For the women in this study, 'their selves were full of duty and obligation generated through their relationships to others rather than legally enforced' (Skeggs 1997:164). Tracey [12] explained this position very clearly:

'You have to do right by your kids don't you? Why else should we bother. Every day I get up and I know that I will struggle to get what they need, feed them, love them, take care of them, it's sort of your duty as a mother isn't it. It's always a struggle, sometimes I nearly go off my head, but it's just what you have to do.'

Phoenix (1991) reports that the women in her study had long anticipated that motherhood would be the most fulfilling aspect of their lives but lack of money was the major problem that most of the women faced. Even those who had partners who earned well in comparison with the rest of the sample reported that they had financial problems. Many in Phoenix's study relied on grandparents for help with meals, clothes and equipment. In 1991, social security benefits were inadequate. In 1999, there had been no change. Being short of money was the major issue for the childbearing women in this study. All had deductions from their income support, to repay previous debts incurred through loans from the social fund or fuel debts. There were no credit unions in Middleton and most women had debts with catalogues, the Provident man or with loan sharks. The main causes of debt were children and Christmas. Children needed clothes and shoes at regular intervals. When household appliances such as washing machines, irons or refrigerators broke down the women found themselves in an impossible situation. The family would be in crisis. On one visit, I asked a woman, Carol [20], why her children were at home and not in school. She said:

'Ryan has no shoes. It is PE today and he has no gym shoes either. I keep him home on PE days and when it's raining. His father says he will get him shoes next week, but he always says that. The Child Support Agency makes him pay £1 a week, that's ridiculous. He says he is not

working, but I know he is, he is on nights in the newspaper, on the delivery lorries. My friend has seen him, he tells them he's not working. He says he can't give the money to the CSA and to me for shoes. He think I can get shoes for £2, the fool.'

It was the lack of money that caused the most distress and prevented her from doing what she saw as best for her child. Carol knew that Ryan ought to go to school but could not do anything about it. The credit offered by major stores, bank loans and credit cards was totally out of the reach of women living in poverty. Yet they still had to prepare for the arrival of a new baby, clothe their children and replace essential household items. None of the women I spoke to had a bank account; some women had tried to open a bank Giro account but they had been refused. Catalogues are an important source of credit and most women had spent up to the maximum they were allowed, around £200. This provided one method of spreading the cost of major purchases but the result was that even more of the fixed weekly income was committed before it arrived. The remainder of the income or the flexible portion was usually that allowed for shopping. The result was that food was the area associated with greatest stress and distress. Getting more credit depended on paying back what was already owed and not being behind with payments. Catalogues were used to purchase toys, prams and other baby equipment as well as clothes and shoes. The Provident man was more flexible; he supplied vouchers that could be exchanged for household goods and school uniforms. He called each week to collect payments of £1 or £2. He was well known in the area and welcomed by the women. The rate of interest varied, but on average a loan of £100 would be repaid by some women at £8 per week for 36 weeks, a total cost of £288. In another example the beliefs about women's responsibilities to their children were expressed by Carol [20]. She said:

'There are a lot of Mums that get into debt and sell their benefit books. It's wrong really because it's the kids money, that £45 belongs to the kids, you should spend it on the kids, but that's the only way to get by really. They will lend on the benefit books.'

The 'loan sharks' were the unofficial moneylenders that operated in the area. All the women told me about the main character; he ran a large fast car and employed a gang of 'strong men' who did the collecting. All women warned against getting involved with him but most had had a loan from him at some stage in their lives. Facts and figures were difficult to obtain but it seemed the rate of interest was around 100 per cent. A loan of £100 had to be paid at the rate of £5 per week; most described how they never repaid the loan but borrowed more as they needed it. One woman, Debbie [15], described how her sister escaped:

'Tina was caught up with J. Every week his blokes called to collect, they wanted £5 but if you could not pay, they would lend you more, you ended up borrowing to pay them. There was never a book or a card, you never knew what you owed or how long there was left to pay. The heavy mob would lean on you, you know insisting you paid, and then they would take the telly and the video. But they were rented ... in the end Tina did a runner ... she left at night and went to Tipton. She lived in a hostel then the Council got her a flat. I don't think they found her, everyone knows about Tina, so they're all a bit wary now.'

Most women received their state benefits with a deduction for rent, council tax and water rates having already been made. The remaining sum had to be used for bills, gas, electric, telephone where one existed, nappies, clothes, food and entertainment. Most women explained that they used their child benefit to pay the catalogue, around £50 per month, used a 'smart card' for the electricity (this is topped up at the local shop), and paid the gas either quarterly or through a meter. Direct debits payments, which attract substantial price reductions, are not available to those without a bank account. Many women had fuel payment arrears; as a result, their income was permanently reduced by deductions to repay the arrears. Paying back debts stretched limited income even further. Those who had a television licence would save using the post office TV savings stamps. One woman, Nikki [11], had a hire purchase agreement for a television set. She said:

'It's a real worry the debt; it makes me feel sick every time I watch it. I want to pay it off quickly.'

Women's responsibilities to their children and the urgency to provide for their children are clearly expressed in the next example. One woman, Tracey [12], summed her position like this:

'I borrow money for school uniforms and for Christmas. The Family Allowance went up but the social took it away. I spend £40 on the food cupboard and £60 in Iceland every fortnight. It's worse in the school holidays. Nappies cost a lot. I spend £500 on Christmas. I have no insurance but I think the council are going to run a scheme for £4.25 a week. I wrote to a trust for some money for school

'uniform, but they said no. I never go out, he has his fishing and the pigeons but I have nothing. The telly is ours, we don't have a licence, the cable is £75 for two months but they are taking that away. I spend £2 on the lottery. I could never work I would lose benefits. I get milk tokens. I smoke 20 ciggies a day that costs £2 from the man in the corner house. I had a drink at my sister's wedding last year. I go to Oxfam and jumble sales. I can't get brand names; a Manchester United kit costs £50 just shorts and a shirt. I borrowed £150 from the Providence man, I repay £4.80 a week, I don't know for how long. The nappies are killing me at the moment [new baby and toddler], Pampers are £6.95 for 45. I always make sure they have clothes to go back to school.'

(Tracey has two children from her first marriage, ages 11 and 9, two from her second, ages 6 and 2, and a new baby.)

There was clear evidence of the so-called 'benefit trap'. Low wages and a lack of permanent posts worked against families in poverty. Jenny [5] explained the position well:

'We get income support and family allowance [child benefit], the rent is stopped out of my money and the council tax, I have to pay gas, electric, water and the phone. I dream about paying the bills. If Morris took a job he would have to earn more than we are getting now. We would have to pay the rent, school meals, and the council tax. What do you do? Morris has been away, you know inside, he can't read or write, the jobs around here just don't pay that sort of money. He's better off helping me when he's here and doing a few foreigners. The social pays people to shop you now, so even that's not worth it.'

The key issues of employment options and low pay are important in considering the ways in which women, and it is mainly their task, manage the money and the household.

Managing the money was probably the most dominating feature of the lives of the women I met with. The task was impossible. All of the women received income support, but over half the women had deductions made for previous debts. As a result, a woman bringing up two children alone has to feed, clothe, furnish the house, pay the heating and other bills on around £85 per week. The week was divided not by a weekend, but by the benefit pay-out day. If the woman received incapacity benefit as well as income support this was paid on a different day and referred to as the Wednesday book and the Monday book. The women referred to their 'paydays' and noted that they often ran out of food and cash before payday. This was especially bad on the weeks when other bills were due, e.g. the electricity, or when the men in their lives had overspent on alcohol or other items considered as luxuries by the women.

A few women felt that they knew and trusted me enough to explain the variety of ways of improving their income. Extra child benefit could be claimed on production of a forged birth certificate but it was recognised that the authorities were more aware of this practice. All the men who were part of the study worked in the 'black economy'. One woman, Nikki [11], said:

'You can get anything you want 'round here. You just have to ask the right person. If you want something doing, someone will do it for the right price.'

And:

'There is a lot of thieving and selling, that's how you get a few bob if you are desperate.'

Tammy [13] said:

'It's easy to get the things you want, you have to know who to ask, the druggies are always looking for things to sell, they will get you what you want. Cheap like, you might have to wait a bit, but they will get it.'

Doing 'a foreigner' was doing any job that paid cash and was not declared to the authorities. Goods were bought and sold via a newspaper called *Bargain Pages* and I was advised that anything I wanted could be acquired. At Christmas time I was offered a computer, a variety of computer games, a Sony Playstation, a Nintendo 64 and a set of fishing rods. No one had household insurance. Burglary, theft and other crimes were commonplace and, according to the women, ignored by the police. Any household goods, toys, games or sporting equipment could be obtained to order. One woman explained, after checking I was nothing to do with 'the social', that her income was boosted by incapacity benefit; her partner had a bad back and was unfit for work, but he was out doing a gardening job when I called. Women derived various strategies to cope with their lives; managing the benefit system to their best advantage was a sensible option. In the midst of debt, financial problems and the strain of poverty it was also important to 'do mothering' well.

Nikki [11] offered this insight into her satisfaction with her role as a mother despite the demands of living in poverty:

'You have to just try to do your best. I want my kids to be the same as everyone else's. I want them to do well in school and have a proper job, even to an apprenticeship. I want them to feel as if I have brought them up right, that I have done my best. They are good kids, they know they can't have everything, but at least they are loved and no one hurts them or nothing. I think that is good. I feel good when I see them all clean in their beds. I know I've done a good job and I am a good mother.'

Foucault (1980) equates this sense of satisfaction with a form of productive power. It is a form of power that comes when women enjoy their responsibilities and where social regulation is achieved willingly by the participants. In this situation, women are not universally oppressed by their responsibilities but derive both power and satisfaction.

SUMMARY

This chapter has set the scene for the study and described something of the environment in which these women lived and brought up their children. It has explored the meaning of motherhood and considered how the middle-class discourses on 'good mothers' and 'good mothering' provide the poor with social codes. It has explored the often contradictory demands placed on women and explored the strong sense of responsibility that these women had towards their children and their childrearing. I have explored some of their motivations for motherhood and examined how motherhood is a route to respectability, a source of happiness and compensation for the hardship of poverty. Finally I have included an example of how motherhood gives some women a sense of satisfaction, a feeling of being respectable and a sense of personal worth.

In the next chapter the themes of respectability and responsibility are continued. The themes are considered in an exploration of social networks, sources of emotional and tangible support and part of the quest for social inclusion.

5

Becoming respectable and sharing responsibilities: grandmothers, networks of support and the search for social inclusion

Introduction
Citizenship and social
  inclusion/exclusion
Categorising the poor
Mothers, daughters, wives and
  husbands

Christmas
Dogs, cats and other animals
Diet, food and shopping
Summary

INTRODUCTION

This chapter explores how individual women with different experiences and backgrounds have different ways of managing their lives as mothers, daughters and as childbearing women living on state benefits. The chapter begins by considering some views on citizenship and social exclusion; it then develops the themes of responsibility and respectability, which were important to the women who contributed to this study. The chapter goes on to explore how some of these women define themselves in relation to other women living in the same locality and explores the meanings of the terms *working poor* and *smelly poor* to these women. The next section briefly explores the concept of social support and examines the ways in which grandmothers were often a crucial part of these women's support networks. It continues the themes of responsibility and respectability by examining how some grandmothers continue to feel a strong sense of responsibility for both their daughters and grandchildren. I use interview data from grandmothers to explore their views on being respectable and to examine how they see changes in life style being equated with a loss of respectability both in individuals and in the locality. I then comment on the difficulties of becoming respectable in an area where the physical environment is declining, and use this to illustrate the scale of difficulties this group of women faced as they lived and brought up their children in Middleton. The next part of this chapter explores more aspects of the culture of this group of women. It gives particular attention to the importance in their lives of Christmas, of keeping exotic pets and how they manage both food and shopping. All these areas of interest are linked by the evidence of the importance of striving for respectability and social inclusion and the strong sense of responsibility this group of women had for their children.

CITIZENSHIP AND SOCIAL INCLUSION/EXCLUSION

For the women in this study, being seen as respectable was very important. The search for respectability is linked with the search for social inclusion. In chapter two, I briefly considered the concept of social inclusion and the setting up of the Social Exclusion Unit as part of the present government's attack on poverty and inequalities in health. As Glendinning and Millar (1992) have shown, access to resources can determine an individual's ability to be a full and active citizen. Citizenship was originally defined by Marshall in 1950 as:

'The right to a modicum of economic welfare and security and to share to the full in the social heritage and to live the life of a civilised being according to the standards prevailing in society' (Marshall 1950:11).

A lack of resources is associated with an inability to participate to the full in society. It results in social exclusion and an inability to exercise all the rights associated with citizenship. By moving house frequently to avoid the bailiffs or simply to avoid paying council tax, women in this study were denied the vote. Moving on was possibly also a way to avoid being sucked into the mire of poverty and desperation. When children went to school hungry or they were kept at home because they had no shoes, they were denied their rights as citizens. Social exclusion prevents citizens from participating to the full in the life of the nation and leaves individuals unable to exercise their rights as citizens.

Charles (2000) argues that poverty diminishes the status of citizenship and because women, along with other minority groups, have access to fewer resources than men, they are more vulnerable to poverty and to a reduction in the status of citizenship. Charles goes on to argue that it is not poverty that reduces the status of citizenship for women but the gendering of citizenship rights which makes women vulnerable to poverty. Social rights of citizenship are based on male patterns of employment. Redefining citizenship so that rights and entitlements are based on unpaid work in the private sphere, the home, as well as paid work in the public sphere is the solution she proposes.

Venanzi (2000) argues that the concept of exclusion has become central in Latin American studies on poverty. The concept has come to replace that of marginality associated with dependency, meaning not only low wages but also a low degree of social and political participation of people living in poverty. Poor people, he argues, are socially excluded from the legal system, because it is inaccessible and expensive; they are excluded from participating in all the benefits of the welfare state, and increasingly from health and education. He believes that in the absence of appropriate political responses, the excluded develop strategies to survive on their own and participate in a very limited way. These views also reflect the assumption that all poor people are the same: it assumes that it is poverty alone that excludes individuals from the legal system, whereas it could be a combination of poverty, lack of knowledge, poor esteem, an inability to articulate complex needs or all of these or any other factors.

Lister (1997) takes a feminist perspective on citizenship. She argues that inclusion and exclusion represent the two sides of the citizenship coin. She examines what she calls the exclusionary tensions inherent in the concept of citizenship and how they operate at different levels to create non or partial citizens; crucially she sees poverty as being corrosive of full citizenship. She is wary of complacency about women's position and is concerned about what she feels feeds the forces of 'post-feminist' backlash in a denial of the extent to which women as a group still enjoy inferior citizenship status. These writers clearly believe that structures are responsible for poverty and the solutions are in the hands of the state. But for these women, universal solutions to universal problems are insufficient. Their lives were complex, multifaceted and very different. They faced their lives and dealt with their problems in different ways. In this study, I was concerned with a small group of 25 women and their relatives; rather than denying the extent of women's inferior citizenship status, I sought to look at the individual consequences. I was particularly interested in the individual effects of poverty and social inclusion. Whilst it is not possible to say that all women are disadvantaged, it is clear that for some women living in poverty, the route to inclusion was frequently hazardous or even blocked.

Being responsible and striving for respectability were important themes throughout this study and some examples of this will be seen later in this chapter. Skeggs (1997) analyses the concepts of respectability and responsibility. She argues that respectability and caring, whilst establishing constraints in women's lives, can be experienced positively. There is evidence of this in chapter two, where these women describe their experiences as mothers and carers as satisfying. This goes some way from the radical feminist position of universal oppression and patriarchal domination and illustrates how women have different experiences and different ways of managing their lives. In this chapter, I explore the views of both the mothers and grandmothers in this area.

CATEGORISING THE POOR

At an early stage in the research, I became conscious that I was seeing two very different types of women in two quite different types of houses. Whilst there were always individual differences there were also similarities and recurring themes. It was in the course of one conversation that a woman referred to herself and her household as '*working poor*'. She described herself as respectable, honest, hard working and doing her best for her children and family. By contrast, she referred to those who lived in other streets as the '*smelly poor*'.

Foucault (1980) uses the term knowledge/power to explain the development of processes of 'normalisation', the techniques and the systems of classification that organise and define deviance and difference. For Foucault, the act of definition and classification is itself an exercise of power. The power is usually associated with universities, research institutions, hospitals, prisons and other socially exclusive institutions such as asylums. However, by defining herself as 'working poor' and others as 'smelly poor', this woman exercised her power. She was able to take up a position of superiority to that of the woman she saw as 'smelly poor'. It could also be that in her interaction with me she felt the need to claim her position in relation to others. Even though I had earned a position of trust and felt that I had the confidence of this group of women, I was still of another class with different values and background. Power, according to Foucault, is exercised not possessed and it has both positive and useful effects. Where there is power there is also resistance. Power is not something that is done to people, something over which they have no control; they are not victims but they use their power to define what they are, describe how they live, and to differentiate them from others.

I was impressed with this woman's definition and once I had heard these terms used, I looked for more evidence and tried to uncover more about these two groups of people; indeed my first task was to see if such a division existed. There was, of course, not a clear-cut division, but it was possible to find a continuum of characteristics and ways of managing poverty. Amongst this group of women, there were some shared common characteristics and values, and in other aspects, there were significant differences in appearance, approach and values. Another woman in this group used the same terms and explored the differences between these two groups in her interview. She was clearly familiar with the language of 'working poor'; she described herself in that way explaining that she had worked as a school-crossing patrol. During the conversation, she made frequent references to the 'smelly poor' as those who lived in another street and whom she considered had poor standards of cleanliness and other antisocial habits. In her opinion, the 'smelly poor' brought down the neighbourhood and led to most families' decision to try to live somewhere else. In asserting herself in this way, this woman was using her knowledge/power to stake her claim as an individual. She did not intend to be labelled as part of a universal group 'the poor' and used the interview with me to claim her difference.

The search for respectability appeared to be peculiar to the 'working poor'.

It appeared that the 'smelly poor' had given up on trying to be respectable. The pressure of poverty had in some way overwhelmed them and left them fighting for the basics for survival. They had no paid employment and lived totally on state benefits supplemented by 'fiddles or foreigners'. Their homes were dirty and unkempt, by my middle-class standards, and by the standards of some of the working poor. The men who were around were intimidating with shaven heads and tattoos; often the men were described as 'away' which I learned was a euphemism for being in prison. Their social networks were different, they reported frequent quarrels with their family, and the women had often lost touch with their own mothers. They all smoked, were frequently survivors of domestic violence, and often drug users and alcohol abusers. They tended to ask for emergency appointments rather than make routine GP appointments and they avoided preventative health services. They resisted the middle-class attempts to 'educate' them by ignoring health advice. They had good relations with social workers whom they saw frequently, and they appeared to get on well with the community midwives. They had very poor housing, often cold and damp with minimal furniture and furnishings. They owned very big dogs and frequently a number of exotic pets. The children appeared to fend for themselves and were regularly suffering from a range of minor illnesses and accidents. Their diet was poor; they often said they were hungry and they always ran out of money every week. Some had sold their benefit books; they looked pale and tired and had few possessions. They had no qualifications, and bought their clothes from jumble sales, the 'tat' man or catalogues. They had never been on holiday, they never voted, they saw education and training as irrelevant and felt they would always manage to survive.

On the other hand, the 'working poor' were striving to be respectable. They sometimes had temporary, part-time, occasional, low-paid jobs. They usually smoked and domestic violence was a common occurrence in their lives. They said that they did not use drugs, and the men used alcohol occasionally. They tended to keep hospital appointments and used preventative health services. They did not usually have a social worker and had good relations with the hospital midwives. They felt it was important to 'pay their way'. Their houses were clean and they took pride in being 'neat and tidy', feeling that to be clean would be a way of gaining respect and the approval of the health-care workers. They sometimes had very large dogs and often had exotic pets. Their diet was poor but they rarely went hungry; they tried hard to manage on what they had and to feel in control. They managed the bills carefully and made sure that child benefit was spent directly on the children. They took pride in their homes; they sometimes had flowers and plants. Some had a few GCSEs; they brought clothes from charity shops, watched videos and had occasional days out at parks. They moved house frequently; they swapped houses to move to better areas. They saw work as the way out of poverty but did not expect much improvement in the quality of their lives until the children were older. They occasionally voted.

These observations are included not to patronise or make judgements about the women who contributed to the study, but to signify the dangers in assuming that there is a single group of the 'poor'. What all these women did share was a struggle to survive life, childbirth and child care on an inadequate income. They coped in many different ways. Even within these two groups, there were differences and individuals making sense of their lives in their own ways.

MOTHERS, DAUGHTERS, WIVES AND HUSBANDS

As part of the investment women make in mothering, most of these women had well-developed links with their own mothers. The grandmothers played a major role in the upbringing of the children and they were a key source of social support and help and guidance to their daughters. The grandmother was frequently the main companion when the woman was in labour. Grandmothers were nearly always present during my interviews and visits. They accompanied their daughters to the antenatal clinics at the GP and at the hospital. They often had a car or had use of a car. Grandmothers always helped with shopping, with child care and with hospital visits. Most of the women in the study saw their own mother every day. They were a constant and main source of support to their daughters as were other female friends and sisters. There was evidence that the relationships that women had with their mothers sometimes influenced their attitudes towards the men in lives and their attitudes to sex, contraception and childrearing. Many of the women in the study had moved house frequently; they often lived some distance from their childhood home and had often lost touch with school friends. Their social networks were frequently built around their mother and their sisters.

The concept of social support first rose to prominence in the 1970s. An American epidemiologist, Lisa Berkman, described it as both preventative and curative medicine. She saw social support as follows:

'Like chicken soup, its powers are believed to be pervasive, the reasons for its effects unknown, and knowledge of its qualities wide spread and based on folk wisdom. ... From interactions amongst mice litter mates to collegiality amongst university graduates, evidence has been garnered to support the notion that social ties are related to good health and well being' (Berkman 1984:413).

Ann Oakley (1992) argues that friendship has been taken to be essentially a personal matter, rather than one which has any social interest or consequence. She notes that a web of classist and sexist assumptions ties the sociological literature on family and community together so that the working classes (especially the women) are seen to rely on kin for social contacts, whilst the middle classes (especially the men) are seen as transcending this primitive dependence and choosing their friends and associates. She argues that conceptually social support overlaps with friendship and both with family, kin and neighbourhood relations. In the medical literature, social support is loosely defined; there are at least 20 instruments for measuring and assessing it in population surveys. It is a complex concept and difficult to define, but includes a wide range of features. It includes such aspects as providing information, nurturance, empathy, encouragement, validating behaviour, constructive genuineness, sharedness, reciprocity, instrumental help, recognition and providing material resources.

Cobb (1976) defines social support as:

'information leading the subject to believe that he [sic] is cared for and loved, esteemed and valued [and] that he belongs to a network of communication and mutual obligation' (1976:300).

Schaefer *et al.* (1981) make a distinction between emotional, tangible and informational support, whilst Kahn and Antonucci (1980) describe affect, affirmation and aid. For those intent on proving cause and effect it is very difficult to measure this elusive concept. When the women in this study talked about the role the mothers played in their lives, family love seemed a clearer concept. They described their mothers in the following ways:

'**Being there, listening, giving me a hug and a fiver,**
Paying the gas bill the day they are going to cut us off,
Looking after the kids when they do my head in,
Bringing a chicken 'round on Wednesday,
Taking us to the park,
Pushing the hoover around when I am tired,
Driving me to the shops,
Staying with me in labour,
Sorting out the DSS and the Housing Department,
Being my friend, listening to my moans,
Being proud of me and being there every day.'

One grandmother was looking after Debbie's children. Debbie [15] said that she was weary; the children were noisy and boisterous. She was around seven months pregnant, had a black eye and was lying on the sofa. She looked pale and very tired. I had met Debbie on a number of occasions; her mother was always with her. Debbie was 19, single and had had five pregnancies. The previous evening she had been attacked by her partner. She explained that they had had a row about money, the children had been very noisy and he had lost his temper. Debbie's partner, Darren, lived with his mother most of the time but was the father of Debbie's children. They had been together for eight years and it had always been a violent relationship. They lived with each other 'on and off'. Debbie introduced Darren to me as 'my hubbie' but later explained that she only said that to people she didn't know, and that as far as the 'social' was concerned she was single. When we first met, she wanted to appear respectable so she said she was married. Debbie said:

'**It's still not proper to be single and have kids. I like to**
pretend I'm married, at least to posh people like you. But I
know you better now ... well anyway. I ain't married and
Darren lives with his mother. That way I get benefits as a
single mother and that suits me well.'

Her mother, Moira, had clear views on the nature of what she saw as 'the problem'. I tape-recorded most of her comments; sometimes the noise from the children obliterated the sound but it was usually possible to fill in the gaps from the field notes. She begins by regretting the changes to the neighbourhood and describing those aspects which have led to its decline. Being respectable is also important to Moira; she regrets that Middleton is no longer respectable. She said:

'**I would like to talk to you. I have lived in Middleton all my life, I have had six children, and I have seen some changes here.**

This used to be a respectable neighbourhood. We moved in in 1960, my husband had work in the leather factory. There was always plenty of overtime in those days. There used to be a bus that picked up the "boys" from the end of the street. People bothered with their houses in those days. The houses belonged to the councils but people treated them like their own. The gardens were always tidy. Everyone had pot plants and hanging baskets.

This area has gone to the dogs now, crime, burglary, and vandals. It's drugs, money to buy drugs. Drugs everywhere you look really. The smack heads are in charge now. They rule the place, that's why everyone wants to get out.' [Moira]

In the next part of the interview, she shares her feelings and thoughts about families and the values of the day. She decries domestic violence and the breakdown of traditional (i.e. married) family life. She believes that women should be more restrained and less liberal. She takes up the theme of responsibility when she talks about men having jobs and providing for their families. This she believes is what men should do.

'**But the real trouble is families. In my day, I would be ashamed to say he lives with me 'on and off'. You got married and stuck by each other, whatever happened. My husband would never lay a finger on me, like that twerp does. He just wouldn't have.**

In my opinion, young girls today are too relaxed with their sexual favours. They are too free and easy with sex. They don't use their wiles. They don't know how to make men respect them. It's there on a plate, they take what they want, knock them about when they get frustrated and disappear back to Mummy.

In the old days there was break. You know, you met a man, waited and then got married. By the time you had sex he was desperate and respected you. We women would withhold sex until they respected us. There's no brake, no holding back now. They meet one day, go to bed the next. No respect. No respect for women, no respect for families. So women like Debbie are just used and abused by men.

And another thing they don't know, the women that is. They don't know how to win them round. You know men like to have a bit of fuss. Like cook him a special meal, that sort of thing. Especially after the baby, they feel left out and then they lash out. Like a toddler really. Women have to know how to handle men to get the best out of them. This generation can't be bothered and it's the likes of me that are left holding the baby.

You see the men are useless. No wages, can't provide. They just don't know how to cope so they knock them about.

If men had jobs and had some sense of responsibility, they wouldn't go away, go back home to their mothers like little boys.

Do you know they don't even have to put their names on the birth certificate now? How will the child feel when they give their birth certificate to someone and it doesn't have their father's name?' [Moira]

Another grandmother had similar views. She felt that it was the loss of the Christian religion that had led to 'the current situation'. Religion was an outward symbol of respectability. When people went to church, they were respectable and the amount of money they had was less important. In the final section of this interview, there is evidence that despite her concerns about the way her daughter and others lived their lives she as a grandmother had a responsibility to her grandchildren. Evelyn said:

'I blame all these immigrants. They all have their religion, you know they go to the Mosque and they wear turbans and that. They don't let their women out. They look after them. The women are modest. Not free and easy with their sexual favours like this lot. Some wear veils, so are all covered up like in a black bin bag. At least they keep themselves pure; they don't treat women like dish rags like these men do.

My grand children know nothing about God. The little one thought Easter was about eggs and said Jesus was killed by Aliens riding on a cross. It breaks my heart really, I brought up my kids to go to Sunday school, dress tidy and have a bit of respect for their elders. It's all gone now, anything goes. Decent people went to church on Sunday, they made an effort.

Now it's sleep with who you like, father kids left right and centre and buzz off. Who's left looking after the kids, granny of course? I can't see the little ones suffer, I have to help out. It's the kids that suffer if I don't. I brought her up right but I don't know what has happened now.'
[Evelyn]

In these extracts, we see examples of how being respectable and taking responsibility were important to grandmothers; these grandmothers regretted that their daughters do not take their advice. They felt that they should make use of their 'woman skills' to make men do what they want them to do. They regret that their daughters have not adopted their ways; they see that 'women's lib' has not liberated their daughters at all. They see them as captive, abused and unsupported by men. The grandmothers used their knowledge/power to get their men to act in a way that was acceptable to them. Their daughters on the other hand used their knowledge and power to escape from some men whom they saw as controlling. Each woman in this study dealt with the demands of her life in poverty in different ways. There were differences between generations and between individual women, but the grandmothers' support and overwhelming responsibility to their children and grandchildren was clearly seen.

How do you become respectable when the environment in which you live is in such poor condition? Middleton was a very deprived area; the nearest park was three miles, a bus ride away. There were no community facilities as such, only the neighbourhood office, which served as a sorting centre for complaints and battles with the housing department. The bus service was infrequent and even the fire brigade required a police escort before it would attend another burning car. The local shops were small, expensive by their standards and the shop windows were frequently boarded up.

The houses all had running water, bathrooms, kitchens and inside toilets but many were damp, with leaking roofs and ill-fitting metal window frames. The bathrooms and kitchens were especially damp with inadequate ventilation. There were no garages but some tenants had cleared a patch in the front garden for a car stand. Some women clearly took a pride in their homes; they were clean, organised and comfortably furnished. Other homes were dirty and poorly equipped. All the homes I visited had colour televisions and video players (a fact confirmed by the 1999 *General Household Survey*). I became quite used to interviewing women around the sound of the television that was always on. The houses were considered by the women to be inadequate. One woman, Judy [17], said:

'I have lived here for eight months; they would not give me a decorating grant so we have had to do it ourselves. My Dad helps me out. There is no central heating, it's freezing upstairs. I have heard that the council are putting in new radiators in every room; touch wood that would be great. There are three bedrooms; the kitchen is like a little galley so we eat on trays. The garden is big but is overgrown, they can't play out there.'

All viewed their stay in Middleton as temporary; they all aimed to move on. Damp, lack of space for children to play, the noise from the neighbours and the high rates of burglary all caused the women additional stress. Some of the houses had central heating but the women worried about the gas bills. Most paid by using tokens in a meter. Some houses had only partial heating in the downstairs rooms, making the upstairs uninhabitable in the winter months. If the heating broke down, the women were dependent on the council to undertake the repairs; the inevitable delays led to frustration and additional stress. Many women felt that their homes were too small; they had nowhere they could go to escape from the constant pressures of caring for the children. One woman said she wanted a shed so that she had a place to go to be alone and have some peace and quiet. One woman, Tracey [12], said:

'It's no wonder kids get battered, if it wasn't for my Mum I'd knock three kinds of shit out of them most days. They are always under my feet, crying, fighting. Making noise. Half term is the worse. In the summer I take them to the park but not in winter. I sometimes think half term was invented to aggravate mothers. You can't send them out to play. The streets aren't safe. They found needles and syringes on the grass last week, last night one of the local lads was taken to hospital in a coma, the drugs are everywhere. The council planted some trees but the older kids vandalised them, now there is nothing. The result the kids are in all the time. If I had the energy I would sort out the garden but it needs too much work and I'm not going to stay.'

Living in Middleton was difficult. These women depended on their mothers to cope and it was difficult for them to see themselves as anything but socially excluded. They lived on the margins of society, endlessly trying to manage and improve the quality of their lives.

CHRISTMAS

In the midst of the difficult times, there was Christmas. Christmas was a very important time for all the women who contributed to this study; it was the one time of the year when they felt they should relax their tight controls over money. The media, television and shops bombarded them with the images of Christmas. Christmas was for children, for families and for self-indulgence; if they had one opportunity to become part of an inclusive society, this was it. They were determined to embrace Christmas in whatever ways they could. Their motivation had its roots in their feelings of responsibility towards their children. Christmas was about giving children a good time and they were determined that their children would be no different from the children they saw on televisions and in films.

I originally avoided any data collection in December; I had thought that this would be a different time and not representative of life in Middleton. I also incorrectly assumed that Christmas would be a non-event and as such not worthy of a period of intensive fieldwork. I was completely wrong. I was to find that Christmas was an important and key conversation topic as early as May. The decorations went up in early November and the packing of presents began in earnest in late November. Nevertheless, Christmas was a worry, a stress and a pleasure for almost half of the year. The women enthused about buying presents, the food and the atmosphere of Christmas. Most women said that they spent around £150 per child on presents. Most felt that Christmas was the only time when borrowing money could be justified. Buying presents for children was the one sure way of proving how much you loved them and how much you cared about their welfare; yet being unable to buy brand names, designer labels and new goods was still a source of stress and distress. The buying begins early in the year. Many women told me of the system whereby a variety of goods could be obtained through dubious means. Following the Christmas of 1998 when certain computer games were very popular, it was possible to arrange a purchase via the 'scam man'. Although I was never sure, I had the impression that various goods were stolen to order.

During my contact with the women of Middleton, I often asked women why they had children; this is explored in chapter four. There were a variety of answers including the need to have someone to love and love them, something to look forward to, the perception that having children would insure against loneliness in old age and the opportunity to do the task of parenting to a better standard than their own parents. All of the women talked about Christmas as a major motivating factor. I noticed that talk about Christmas was animated and led to enthusiasm and excitement as the women talked. One woman, Barbara [10], seemed to confirm all that the others had said. She said:

'Christmas is a really special time. We plan for it all year, it's what it's all about really. I spend a lot, I start buying in July or August, I put the tree up once the clocks go back in October, around half term. Every year I buy more decorations and another set of lights. Last year I had four trees, two were artificial but two were real. They sell them off really cheap on Christmas Eve. We have a turkey, sweets, a ham, crackers, biscuits. The telly, but no one watches that. I start buying extra food as soon as it comes into the shops. Aldi starts when the clocks go back. It's the one chance to go over the top, you know let your hair down. I can do it because it's for the kids. It shows them that I really love them, then they love me too. I couldn't not do all that. How else would you show them you love them?

Last year they were so excited they didn't go to bed until 5 a.m. It's seeing their faces when they open the presents,

that makes it all worthwhile. The babby won't notice much this year, just play with the wrapping paper like he did last year. But once they get to two they get wound up like the rest of them. It is really the most important thing; I'd do anything to get them what they want. I did one year, I went on the game to buy presents. It's easy money really, £30 a go, but I got sick of it. I hated being used, but it was worth it to see them open their presents.'

Another woman described Christmas like this:

'Christmas is what it's all about really. When they are grown up and have kids of their own, I'll be a grandmother and go and visit them. They will do it like I do. You know the tree, presents, turkey and that. What happens to them now they will remember, it's really important. I could not bear them to think back and feel it was terrible. I want them to think of Christmas as the best time. The struggle in January, and February, and March goes away, it's Christmas they remember.'

Most of the women who contributed to this study (all except one) were just about managing to cope with their poverty but Christmas was an important and completely necessary expense. Christmas was a time to show they loved their children, that they cared for them, that they placed their needs over and above their own. Children were their responsibility; they were even responsible for their children's memories. They 'did' Christmas because they were driven by the responsibilities of parenthood. In embracing Christmas they were the same as everyone else. The media would have us believe that spending excessively at Christmas is a sure and certain route to happiness. It is essential and the effort involved entirely justified: for the rich and the poor to make Christmas a priority is part of being part of an inclusive society.

DOGS, CATS AND OTHER ANIMALS

During the fieldwork stage of this research, I quickly had to adapt to the practice of keeping pets. I did not realise that keeping a pet was such an important aspect of the lives of the women. In a way, it was one of the features of my culture shock; I hated animals, in particular big dogs that jumped up at me. It was the one factor that led me closest to giving up the study. The women could see my fear; sometimes they would lock the dog outside, but other times they just laughed at me. Out of 35 homes I visited, I found the following.

Dogs	Cats	Rabbits/Hamsters	Other Exotic Pets
25	18	32	25

The exotic pets were the most intriguing. These included snakes, iguanas, lizards, and other reptiles, e.g. 'hooded dragon', rats, spiders and locusts. My interview with Barbara [10] was a typical example. In response to my question, 'Tell me about your pets?', she said:

'I have a bearded dragon in the tank over there, a hooded rat, he's quite poorly at the moment, he's got cancer, the tumour is on his back. A mouse called Trevor, he won't come out if he knows there is someone in the room. A hamster called Frank he lives in the kitchen. Two rabbits outside called George and Mildred. They are three quarters angora. I don't know what the other quarter is. I have two dogs, Pekinese cross. There are stick insects breeding in that glass, they are to feed the hooded dragon. I have a frog in the bedroom, and a lizard in the tank. I used to have a snake but it grew too big for the tank so I got the RSPCA to take it away. I want tropical fish but I can't afford a tank just yet.'

Figure 5.1 is a diagram of her living room. It was very difficult to move in such a small room; the smell from the pets was overpowering and it was obvious that the pets were very important to Barbara and her family. At the end of one conversation Barbara said, 'I am going to get a Bison, the health visitor says I have to.' I was alarmed and had visions of a large cow occupying the remaining space in the small living room. However, I had misunderstood her comment; she had said she was going to get a Dyson (a vacuum cleaner). I asked why she had so many pets. She said that she liked looking after things: it was something to love, her partner did not live with her all the time and she was lonely. As a child she was not allowed any pets; now she loves having them around. She also felt that her three children, and a new baby, would benefit from having pets. She did not want them to miss pets as she had done as a child. The health visitor had warned of the dangers of letting pets out in the same room as a new baby but she dismissed her advice as irrelevant.

I considered the significance of pets in women's lives. Was it, in an environment of deprivation, a symbol of difference and an opportunity to mark out your individuality? I dismissed this explanation; so many women had pets that to have them was not being different. It may have been more about conforming and being the same as others. The pets were expensive and the equipment needed to look after them was expensive but that was not an issue. Dogs were treated at the RSPCA even though this meant finding someone to take them to a neighbouring town for treatment. They usually found a parent who would give them a lift. I believe that their sense of responsibility extended to their pet animals. It was part of the power that comes with responsibility and a sense of satisfaction of having achieved something. Having a very unusual pet was also part of being different; it was a clear way of marking yourself apart from the crowd. One woman kept a python; this snake was very large and its existence well known in the neighbourhood. It was kept in a glass tank in the living room. The midwives warned me about it, the other women discussed it and it was clearly a source of pride for its owner. In a life dominated by struggle, poverty and distress, the snake was a source of pleasure and pride. Having pets and even exotic pets was not unusual in Middleton. It was not seen as different; it was simply what the people around there did.

Figure 5.1: Barbara's living room

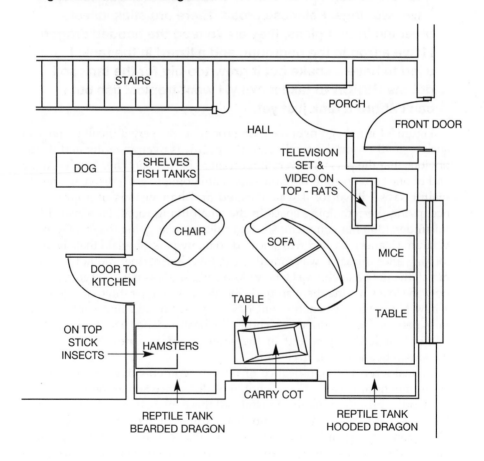

DIET, FOOD AND SHOPPING

In ethnographic research, the researcher has very little control over the issues that present. The researcher may begin with ideas or foreshadowed problems but the issues arise unexpectedly. Throughout the research, it became clear that buying food, going shopping, making the food last and conforming to the pressures to provide their children with a 'balanced diet' were very important issues for these women.

I entered the field without a clear plan of the issues I wanted to discuss. I wanted to understand how childbearing women living in poverty made sense of their lives and experiences. The women I met wanted to talk about food and providing for their children. As mothers, providing food for their children was an important part of their responsibilities. I did not try to draw definitive conclusions about the quality of either their diet or its nutritional content but it was possible to assess attitudes to diet and to food and learn more about how each woman coped with the struggle to make ends meet.

Anne Murcott (1998) argues that food is more than just something to eat. She writes:

'Eating does more than keep the human organism going (or fail to do it). Food brings the natural and the social (in its generic sense i.e. To include the economic, psychological, cultural) into focus. Eating serves as one means of describing the manner in which human beings are simultaneously biological organisms and social beings ... food means more than biological survival; it also means psychological and cultural survival, and is some of the stuff of social and economic relationships' (1998:14).

It is against this backdrop that this section must be considered. For these women living in poverty and coping with an inadequate income, food is more a source of pain than it is pleasure. Dawn [16] summarised her position like this:

'You just have to be very, very careful. All the time. You can manage if you are a tight arse. Find a cheap butcher, go to the market, if you can walk that far or have the money for the bus fare. Shop very carefully. Apples can be 20p in one shop, 50p in another. Buy what you need no more everything else is a luxury. I go to the shops nearly every day; I buy the bargains and get what we need. Nothing more, nothing less.

Baby stuff is cheap, hand me downs for clothes, and avoid the traps like catalogues. Iceland, Aldi and Netto are okay if you can get a lift, but they all make you spend too much. If you go to the shops on Saturday just as they are closing,

there are some bargains then. But all the shops make you spend too much.'

Food, calorie intake and diet have interested survey researchers for many years. How to solve the 'problems' of the poor and how to get them to do a better job of feeding their children have been dominant issues in social and health research. Once again, there is a search for a universal solution. Dowler and Calvert (1995) carried out a cross-sectional survey of 200 lone-parent households in Greater London. Data were obtained from individual three-day weighed intake records for each parent and at least one child. They also used a food frequency questionnaire, and a taped semi-structured interview. The results indicated that poor material circumstances combined with severe constraints on disposable income were the main factors characterising nutritional deprivation in lone parents and sometimes their children. They said:

'Parents who lived for more than a year in local authority or privately rented housing, who were unemployed, had had no holiday, had had fixed, regular deductions from a low budget consistently had markedly lower intakes of nutrients and patterns of diet that were less healthy than parents who were not living under these circumstances' (1995:36).

They also found that children's diets were less varied in the poorest households, and vitamin C intakes were lowest. Parents claiming income support had worse micronutrient and iron intakes than those who did not claim it. Smoking made no difference and the further from benefit collection day, the worse the diets. These authors demonstrated that those who live in the poorest conditions could not afford to eat healthily. Automatic deductions from the benefit system for arrears and debts meant that many of their respondents could not afford the food they needed.

In this study, all of the women were pregnant or were in the early postnatal period. Pregnancy places additional demands on the body. To grow healthy babies, women need a good diet and sufficient calories. In 1995, the Maternity Alliance, a pressure group campaigning to improve the life of pregnant women, new parents and their babies, published *Poor Expectations* and claimed that a healthy balanced diet was impossible to achieve on state benefits. They demonstrated that the type of diet recommended to woman in antenatal clinics would take up 39 per cent of the income of a single 25 year old on income support and 49 per cent of the income of a pregnant 18-24 year old. The major concern about diet before and during pregnancy is its possible link with low birth weight. Low birth-weight babies are at greater risk of a range of health problems, and the effects may last through childhood and into adulthood.

In another study undertaken by Rothwell (1995), it was found that childbearing women on low incomes did not try to follow advice on diet; some saw the advice as inconsistent and inappropriate and the experience of physical problems was the only incentive for following advice. Foods were considered to be 'healthy' in proportion to how much they were believed to alleviate physical discomforts or to achieve a desired body size. Support from the extended family appeared to protect women from the stress of managing on a low income but it did not seem to improve the nutritional quality of the diet of some women. In Rothwell's study the pooling of resources amongst relations seemed to cushion women's diets from the harsher effects of low income. Such studies are useful in informing governments and others that it is difficult to eat a healthy diet on benefits. Rather than offering blanket solutions, what is interesting is looking at the ways in which individual women coped with these difficulties.

In this study, many of the women would have been in difficulty if they had not had regular and frequent contact with their mother or mother-in-law. Many women relied on their mothers and would visit them frequently; the visit always included a meal. In this study, all of their children had free school meals and all of the women were in receipt of state benefits; free meals and milk tokens were very important. School holidays and weekends meant an extra burden in that the women had to find extra meals for hungry, growing children. One woman, Dawn [16], described how she fell out with her mother but made friends because the children needed her mother's dinners.

Some women were willing to describe their 'stock cupboards'. These contained very little food; what was bought was eaten and there was very little in the cupboard that could be made into a meal. The children appeared to 'graze', often eating crisps and biscuits throughout the day. Debbie [15], a 19-year-old mother of three children and pregnant, explained:

'I try to tell them "when it's gone it's gone", but they don't understand. The cupboards are empty, we try to manage until payday, but sometimes on Wednesday there is just nothing. I send them to my Mam's sometimes she gives them a dinner. I go without, I am always trying to lose weight, but it never helps. I drink hot tea and that fills me up. You get sick to death of asking the butcher for bones for the dog and making soup. One day I am going buy really posh food like steak or fish or even a vegetable like a courgette.'

Kirsty [21] explained how she dealt with the difficulties of providing her children and herself with an adequate diet:

'I get sick to death with the midwives at the hospital. They go on and on about eating liver and green leafy vegetables. I hate liver; I haven't eaten it since I was a kid.

And if I buy cabbage or greens I end up throwing it out, so that's a waste. It's much better to buy what the kids will eat, at least then it's not wasted. Sometimes I buy myself an orange, it's good for the new baby. I heard this thing on the telly about diet, they can't make their minds up can they. One day eggs are no good, one day it's meat that's bad. I make my own mind up, tell them at the clinic what they want to hear and take the iron tablets when I feel like.

The kids are growing, I go hungry not them, that is the proof I need. Of course more money would help, I'd buy more treats I think, vegetables are okay, we have sprouts at Christmas and eat lots of potatoes, so what's the problem?'

The women in this study were not victims, they did what they could to survive, they did their best and made sure that their children came first. They resented being labelled as inadequate by health professionals and being offered standard advice with no concern for them as individuals.

Wynn *et al.* (1994) recorded and analysed the diets of 513 London mothers. These authors concluded that although there was no social gradient for total calorie intake there was a statistically highly significant social class gradient for intake of protein, seven minerals and six B vitamins, all of which are highly significantly correlated with birth weight. Doyal *et al.* (1991) argue that although improvements in maternal diet may achieve an increase in birth weight, better results are achieved if the diet is improved before conception. If the diet is consistently inadequate, this has little relevance. Carbohydrate and fatty foods are relatively inexpensive but fresh food, green leafy vegetables, folic acid enriched bread and other enhanced cereals are beyond the reach of women living on state benefits. Improving the diet before conception involves a degree of planning and forethought; offering advice that fails to take into account individuals' life styles and motivations often becomes irrelevant.

It appears that it is women who control the food purchasing and consumption in most households. Women decide what to buy and what to leave on the supermarket shelf. Women go without if the money is more than usually tight, and women make the decision on what will be left out if an unexpected bill arrives. These women controlled what was eaten in a family and some went without if the food was short; being pregnant made no difference. The women were never able to entertain at home or eat out in a restaurant or cafe; take-away foods were limited to fish and chips, and buying new or different foods was too risky in case the children did not like the food and it was wasted.

SUMMARY

This chapter has continued the exploration of some aspects of the culture of Middleton and an examination of the lives of this group of women as they live, become pregnant, have children and rear those children whilst surviving on inadequate state benefits. They do this whilst living in a very poor environment, with dismal housing and inadequate local facilities. In particular, it has given attention to how individuals face the difficulties of poverty. It has considered how women as a group were compromised and socially excluded as citizens. It has continued the themes of responsibility and respectability and examined these in relation to the definitions of themselves, to social support and to the role of grandmothers. It has examined the importance of Christmas and the significance of exotic pets, and the realities of managing food and shopping on an inadequate income. This chapter has provided the rich descriptive data of an ethnographic study, but rather than describing a homogeneous culture, there is an attempt to see these aspects from the perspective of individuals. The aim has not been to make generalisations about all childbearing women living in poverty or to offer universal solutions. Whilst it is clear that an increase in state benefits and the abolition of fuel debts would certainly help most women, the aim is not to solve the problem of pregnancy and poverty. The aim has been to understand more of the complexities of these women's lives and take another step towards understanding the impact of poverty on individual women. In this chapter, we have seen the variety of ways in which these women deal with poverty, and the complexities that surround the social distress of poverty. These women lived with poverty; there were common themes but also differences in the ways in which they approached their lives and coped with their distress. O'Brian and Penna (1998) emphasise the need to shift away from universal prescriptions for alleviating social distress and to emphasise the multiple agenda which any welfare programme generates.

The next chapter considers in more detail the relationships that these women had with the men in their lives. Having become a feminist in the 1980s, I expected the women to be oppressed and victims of the structure that supported them. However, as the theoretical framework of this thesis veered towards a poststructural one, like Braidotti (1991) I realised the significance of 'Foucaultlacanderrida' in shaping my understanding of how I perceive other women and how women perceive themselves. Such complex investigations into the subjectivity of a sense of self meant that I had to abandon the 'truth claims' that dominated feminist activism in the 1980s and instead listen to the interpretations of the women in the study. These women believed that they were strong and revealed their 'sense of self' (Stacey 1997) through language and a clear determination to do right by their children. Far from being victims, these women appeared to be strong and able to make decisions about their lives and future.

6

Strong women and restless men

INTRODUCTION

This chapter explores the changing and varied nature of the relationships between childbearing women living in poverty in the West Midlands and the men who are 'in and out' of their lives. In my research, I found what seemed to be a recurrent and common understanding of the role of men in some women's lives; there were similarities in the ways in which they described men. Those men without paid employment were referred to in terms such as: '*No wage, and no use*'. It seemed to me that these men were dismissed as irrelevant when they failed to be breadwinners and economically active. However, this apparent dismissal of men was sometimes contradicted. Some women were driven by the need to conform to the respectable image of the family and to be married with 'two point two children'. For them the phrase '*any man is better than no man*' was more dominant. It seemed that to be with a man, any man, even a man who had no job, was better than being a single mother. In this chapter, I explore the different ways in which women come to terms with what appeared to me to be unstable and dissatisfying relationships with men. Initially I saw these women as victims of men's behaviour but, in fact, many were more survivors than victims; some were very strong, resilient and single-minded. Most were dedicated to the care of their children and determined to carry on with or without men. Throughout the study, I was conscious of women's need and urgency to gain control over their lives but they achieved this goal in different ways. Some were clearly disillusioned by the inadequacies of their '*restless men*', but they were willing to trade the promise of emotional and physical support for peace and control over their own lives, and for stability. They seemed to build their support networks around other women, mainly their own mother, and chose to exclude men who let them down, abused them and failed to provide for them either physically or emotionally. Other women described how they made the best of a bad job. They described how, despite the difficulties of their relationship with men, they stayed in the relationship. To be seen as respectable and conforming was clearly important. Therefore, despite the rapidly changing nature of the society around them, some women used their own power to make the best of what was on offer. Whilst many women said that they wanted a happy family life, a nice home, a big garden, and a loyal man who was a good provider, when it became obvious to them that all these things were unavailable, they made the best of what they had.

In the first section, I will reiterate some of the explanations of unemployment and the impact of unemployment on women. I will briefly explore the ways in which health professionals and midwives in particular fail to recognise the complexities of women's relationships and households. In the next section, I will examine the changing nature of households and families as seen in official government reports and research papers. I will then explore some of the complex family structures I observed and draw on conversations with women to illustrate the complexities and differences in their life styles and relationships. I use Rachel's [2] words to explore the theme of 'weighing up the costs and going it alone'. I build on this example to explore the link between effective parenting and having sufficient resources. Rachel found that not only was living alone better for her, but it enabled her to manage her resources more effectively. It also gave her the freedom and power to be a better parent. Kirsty's [21] story is used to illustrate the tensions between looking for support from men and the decision to live alone. Despite her need for a man for support, she lives alone (with her children). She has gained a measure of control and exerted power over her life.

In the next section, I describe Paul and his relationship with both Jenny [5] and Sharon [9]. Jenny uses the term '*putting up and putting off*' to describe her relationship with Paul. She wants the respectability and stability of a close relationship but she knows that it is unobtainable. She exercises her power and 'puts off' the decision to leave him and live alone with her children.

I then consider Sarah [8], a 15-year-old woman who was in the late stages of an unplanned pregnancy when I first met her. She concluded that men were a 'waste of time'. The man who was the father of her child had no wage and was therefore, in her opinion, of no use. She had learned to survive with the support of her mother and her sisters and not the support of a man. I next consider Joanna [22] who opted to live with her partner Trevor. They concluded that living together was the best option for them. Finally, I draw on my many conversations with Claire [24]. Claire was an older and more experienced woman who explained how she felt that for her there was no other option but to live apart from men. Whilst being a mother on her own was a struggle she felt that men did not fit into her life any more. She had given up on being respectable and felt she was 'okay' and more in control alone. She saw clearly that her role was in socialising her boys to become better men, husbands and fathers.

WHY 'NO WAGE, NO USE'?

The economic structures of the UK exert a significant influence on men and subsequently on their ability to act as providers to the household. The West Midlands was previously the centre of the English manufacturing industry; however, in 1996 the unemployment rate for Middleton was more than 20 per cent. Unemployment rates nationally are highest amongst young adults. According to *Social Trends 28* (ONS 1998b), in the spring of 1997 nearly one fifth of all economically active 16-19-year-old men, and nearly a seventh of women of the same age, were unemployed. Generally the less a person is qualified the greater the chance of being unemployed.

In the government's later report which monitors poverty, *Monitoring Poverty and Social Exclusion 2001* (Rahman *et al.* 2001), in its chapter on young adults it is stated that the unemployment rate amongst young adults is significantly higher than for adults over 25. Unemployment is a major cause of low income and deprivation. The report's authors see the first barrier to work as a lack of educational qualifications. The indicators in this report show that large numbers of young adults remain economically vulnerable. The structural responses include 'New Deal' and the introduction of the national minimum wage. The Rahman report acknowledges that low pay remains a major problem in young adults and that there are still 150,000 young adults who are not in education, training or work. A quarter of the age group currently lack a basic qualification (NVQ2 or equivalent) and a tenth lack any form of qualification. It is no surprise therefore that in 1999-2000 the numbers on low incomes remain at a historic high. At least 150,000 pupils each year still fail to obtain any GCSEs above grade D, and 25,000 still get no grades at all.

The men in this study were poorly qualified, many had left school at the first opportunity and they had few skills. The government's 'New Deal' policy is aimed at improving the employability of the long-term unemployed and those on benefits so as to help them into jobs. It is aimed at four groups, the first of which is 18-24 year olds who have been claiming Job Seekers Allowance for six months or more. Other groups include lone parents, mainly women, for whom there are now greater job opportunities and supported child care.

There was a strong feeling amongst the women I interviewed, and their mothers, that the men in their lives lacked maturity. The women told me that the men would not stick to poorly paid, repetitive jobs in the local factories. Whilst the men in the study lived with the women who were the mothers of their children 'on and off', they frequently went home to their own mother if things became difficult. They had little experience of taking responsibility; they frequently had no work. They were generally lacking basic educational qualifications and, at the time of the study, they had limited opportunities to acquire training or join apprenticeship schemes.

This study focuses on childbearing women living in poverty. I did not choose to study men, neither did I take time to explore the effects of unemployment on men and their relationships. This is for others. There is no doubt that the men were deeply affected by the economic situation and by their lack of well-paid, continuous employment. These issues had an impact on their lives and on the lives of their wives, girlfriends and partners. My concern with men was limited to the impact their actions and life styles had on individual women in the study and the choices that they made. It could also be argued that young men have an unrealistic idea of the nature of relationships with women. Based on *Neighbours, Home and Away* and other soap operas, young men have little idea of what is needed to sustain a relationship. On the other hand, the women are faced with the physical, emotional and psychological demands of motherhood and are forced to mature quickly and take the responsibility of a new baby as soon as it arrives. The media portrayals of motherhood are also unrealistic: smiling, sweet-smelling babies who sleep for long periods in the arms of doting parents are a long way from the reality.

In this study, I was also interested in the nature of the relationship between childbearing women and midwives. I knew that health-care professionals had a range of euphemistic titles for pregnant women who were not married and were living outside 'normal' traditional family relationships, but the notes simply reflect single, married or divorced. These categories failed to reflect the complexity of childbearing women's relationships with the men in their lives and failed to recognise the impact that such relationships or lack of them may have on the pregnancy outcomes. Professionals frequently fail to acknowledge the differences in women and women's lives. These issues are explored in more detail in chapter eight. The women in this study were part of society and the structure of society itself has changed quite significantly in recent years. Structures are more fluid, and individuals' positions in those structures are less likely to be fixed or customary. The traditional family with a married mother and father and their two children has changed significantly in recent years both in Middleton and in the UK.

THE CHANGING NATURE OF HOUSEHOLDS AND FAMILIES

According to information presented in *Social Trends 31* (ONS 2001:43), the so-called 'nuclear' or 'traditional' family household consisting of a couple living in their own home has been predominant since at least the late sixteenth century. Household composition, however, has transformed in recent decades. More people live alone, and the proportion of couple family households with dependent children fell from two fifths in 1961 to less than a quarter in 2000. The proportion of lone-parent households with dependent children has tripled. In spring 2000 one in ten people in Britain lived in a lone-parent household.

A family is legally defined as a married or cohabiting couple, with or without their never-married children who have no children of their own, or a lone parent with such children. There has been a substantial growth in the number of lone-parent families; most are headed by a lone mother. In 1996, 21 per cent of all families with dependent children were headed by a lone parent. Divorce provides some of the explanation for the rapid rise of lone-parent families, but after the mid-1980s the number of single lone mothers grew at a faster rate than the proportion of births outside marriage. The 1980s saw a growing separation of marriage and childbearing, with one in three children being born outside marriage.

COHABITATION IN THE 1990s

Social Trends 28 (ONS 1998b) also reports the fall in the proportion of people living as married couples and the increase in cohabitation. The 2001 edition of *Social Trends 31* (ONS 2001) notes that the pattern of partnership formation has changed since the mid-1970s and although the majority of men and women still get married, that majority is not quite as large as it was. The proportion of men and women who are marrying has been declining, the proportion cohabiting has been increasing and the proportion living outside a partnership has also increased. The proportion of all non-married women aged 18-49 who were cohabiting in Great Britain has doubled since 1981 to 25 per cent in 1996-97. The proportion of single women cohabiting increased from 9 per cent in 1981 to 27 per cent in 1996-97. The rise in divorced women cohabiting has been small in comparison; the proportion increased from 20 per cent to 32 per cent over the same period. Cohabiting implies a relationship where people of the opposite sex live together as a prelude or as an alternative to marriage. It is certainly correct to state that the type of family in which a child grows up has changed over the past 30 or so years. There is a decrease in the percentages of dependent children living in couple families and an increase in those living in lone-parent families but the traditional couple family still remains the most common type of family in which children live (*Social Trends 31*, ONS 2001).

Keirnan and Estaugh (1993) claim that cohabiting prior to marriage is now a majority practice: around seven in ten remarriages are preceded by a period of cohabitation. Cohabiting unions tend to be short-lived, around two years on average, and either convert into marriages or break up. In this study, four women described themselves as cohabiting and 11 as single; sometimes they used the term cohabiting even if they were 'cohabiting' for only one or two days per week.

The *British Social Attitudes* survey (Jowell *et al.* 1990) investigated attitudes to cohabiting and revealed that four out of ten respondents would advise a period of premarital cohabitation before marriage; only 18 per cent of under-35 year olds would advise a couple to marry without living together first. Similarly, attitudes to having children outside marriage were considered; 73 per cent of men and 68 per cent of women agreed that people who want children should get married, but in the under-25s respondents group (the age group most likely to be having children) less than one half thought that people who want children ought to become married.

Kiernan and Estaugh (1993) consider that the trend to live together before marrying may well become an institutionalised part of the mating process, in the same way as engagement was in the past. Only a minority of cohabiting couples has dependent children: one in four of the never-married cohabiting group. Using information from the *General Household Survey*, they found that cohabiting couple families were more likely to be in receipt of income support and housing benefit, to be in local authority accommodation, and the male partner was more likely to be unemployed or be a semi-skilled or unskilled occupation than is the case in married couple families. They concluded, 'that on most of the available measures, the cohabiting couple with children were less well-off than their married counterparts' (1993:17).

According to *Social Trends 31* (ONS 2001) one-parent families tend to be more vulnerable than couple families, whether from the point of view of economic deprivation, greater health problems or general social disadvantage. These are the statistics and the observations made on the basis of scientific calculations; in the midst of these facts and figures are individuals who 'buck the trend' or who just do not quite match up to the statistics. In the data that follows it is possible to see the person behind the figures: the Tracey, the Barbara and the Sharon. It is too easy to categorise people and make erroneous assumptions about their life styles and circumstances.

The social security system treats cohabiting couples as if they were married (which is possibly why so many women reported themselves as single, even though they were living in a relatively stable relationship with one man). The taxation authorities treat cohabiting couples as two separate and distinct individuals. Taxation and inheritance laws are still based on the assumption that women are dependent on their spouses. The legal system is acknowledging the change and recognises relationships outside marriage. As a minimum, the law recognises the contributions towards the purchase of a family home and its contents and the right to live in a home free of violence. Kiernan and Estaugh (1993) conclude their study of cohabitation by saying, 'it is likely that many people cohabit without seriously informing themselves about the consequences of not marrying'.

In the next section, I will explore some of the family structures that I observed and I will draw on conversations with some women to illustrate the complexities and differences of their life styles and relationships. In this study initially only four women out of 25 described themselves as married. As I became more familiar with the women and they grew to trust and accept me, they changed the descriptions of their status. Some of those who had previously described themselves as married later said that they were cohabiting but felt that married was more acceptable to the 'lady researcher' from the university. It is not surprising that I appeared to represent the 'upper classes'. They had no reason to trust me; they were not sure at first if I represented the social services or the social security system. Some felt that I was 'snooping' and would report them to a variety of agencies. It took time to build relationships in the field and it took time for the women to trust me and share aspects of their lives with me. There is no doubt that at first I was surprised or even shocked by the nature of their relationships. It took time for me to stand back and reflect on the differences between my life style and those I was observing. I acknowledged my weaknesses and took steps to change my body language, appearance and attitudes. I did not always succeed, but as the study progressed, I felt that I was amongst friends who were willing to help me and whom I was willing to help. I cannot claim that I achieved unconditional positive regard, which is my personal philosophy in midwifery care, but I certainly achieved respect and admiration for the women and how they coped with the day-to-day difficulties of their lives.

Rachel's story was a good example of these complex family groups. The following is my field note for my first visit. A diagram, Figure 6.1, helps to explain the scene.

'Rachel [2] originally described herself to me as married, but today, my third meeting with her, she says that she is divorced, cohabiting or separated from Alfie. Rachel has three children: there are Amy and John, she is divorced from their father, John, but sees and cares for the daughter of his first marriage, Kelly, on a regular basis. Her third child, Sarah, was born soon after she met Alfie, who now lives with her on and off. Rachel cares for Amy, John, Kelly [the child born from her husband's first marriage], Sarah and she is expecting her fourth child in four weeks.

Amy and John's Dad, also John, was a "disaster", he smoked, drank heavily and "knocked her about a bit". He would not drink tea or coffee; only Coke or Pepsi and this at £1 a bottle became a huge drain on the family's meagre income. He also ran a car that required petrol and frequent repairs. Rachel described how no matter what she did, she would always run out of money before the next payday. She then decided to divorce John and Amy's father, and soon met up with Alfie. She said that after the divorce she coped much better. At first she wanted to live with Alfie, but she felt that she was doing so much better on her own. Alfie has a job so if he were to move in she would lose milk tokens, free school meals, council tax, and free prescriptions and have to start paying rent. She would have to claim family credit and that just would not be worth it. Alfie is a long distance lorry driver and has a daughter from a previous relationship and visits her at weekends.' [Field Note]

Figure 6.1

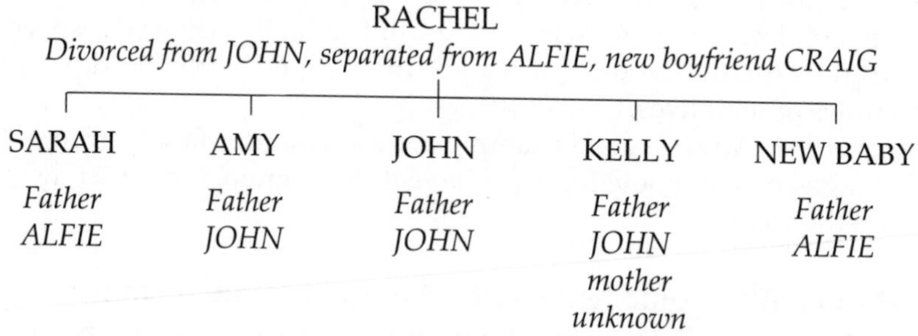

RACHEL
Divorced from JOHN, separated from ALFIE, new boyfriend CRAIG

SARAH	AMY	JOHN	KELLY	NEW BABY
Father	*Father*	*Father*	*Father*	*Father*
ALFIE	*JOHN*	*JOHN*	*JOHN*	*ALFIE*
			mother	
			unknown	

WEIGHING UP THE COSTS AND GOING IT ALONE

Rachel's analysis of the costs and benefits of a relationship with Alfie are particularly important. Having been bruised by her relationship with John, the father of her first two children, she had learned that she was able to manage far more effectively on her own. At 22 years of age, she was caring for four children and expecting her own fourth child in the near future. During the course of our meetings, she reflected on her life and on her decisions. She said:

'When I was pregnant I felt I really needed him [John], but apart from taking me shopping he didn't do much at all. I was pregnant, I would be on my hands and knees when the vacuum cleaner broke, cleaning the carpets with a dust pan and brush. He would just sit there watching TV.

He could get up and help ... I would cook for him every night; he did not help to wash up, even if I was tired. He would be in a mood, if he had not had a good week he would not give me anything. I would tell him I was tired, some weeks he would give me a bit of extra money for his food. Even when he didn't give me money I could cope but that's not it. I have been waiting for him to push the washing machine back under the surface for weeks; I have to pull it out to hook the pipe over the sink, now I do it myself. It's getting difficult with the bump getting bigger but I manage. Sometimes he would say 'you are pregnant, I'll do it', but if a job lasted more than ten seconds he would not do it. I can get a taxi to the shops. I always have money in my purse now, not like when I was married. If I stay single things will get a lot better. It's being with a man that causes all the problems; it's just not worth it. I love my kids and I'll do all right by them. Alfie is no better than John, he can't stand Amy or John, he gets cross with Sarah, they are just normal kids. Getting his dinner every night is no good, I can't feel in control when he is there. It's just not worth the trouble.

Having almost given up on men in her life, Rachel is in the process of building a life without a close relationship with a man. She has exchanged what has been minimal emotional and physical support for peace, control over her money and the opportunity to build her own life. In this example, Rachel makes it clear that, for her, life is better on her own. She feels that she has greater control of the family's income and consequently she is better able to provide for her children. However, she is faced with the discourses that claim she is an inadequate mother, because she is single. The media argues that she is feckless, worthless and a drain on society's resources. In fact, in this case it is the man who is a greater drain on her resources and the resources provided by the country. She has worked out for herself that she is better off without a man despite the pressure to conform. As a mother who has chosen to live alone she has better control of the family income and can make better decisions about how to meet the family's needs.

In this case, we see that a young, single mother risks greater financial insecurity if she stays with a man. On her own she retains power and control over money, over her children and over the domestic environment. In fact, she manages more effectively. The downside to this arrangement is that she loses respectability. She loses the respect of a society that is essentially patriarchal; it assumes that women need a man to care and provide for them.

In this case the opposite applies; when Rachel was in a relationship her dependency on the state increased and she was in greater danger of having her children put into care. She concluded that she was better off on her own. For midwives this is an interesting example of how it is quite easy to make assumptions and presume that Rachel fits a classic stereotype. It would take more time than most midwives have to unravel the complexities of Rachel's life and to understand her motivations, incentives and decisions. Individualised care requires some measure of understanding of where Rachel is now and what issues are important to her in the future.

In Ferri and Smith's 1996 study of parenting in the 1990s, based on data collected as part of the National Child Development Study, the researchers discovered that successful parenting required adequate resources. Parents needed sufficient income to provide a satisfactory material environment; they needed time as well as the personal qualities appropriate to meeting their children's needs for emotional security, stability and affection. These researchers also found that a sizeable minority of parents, especially mothers, were not happy with their marriage relationship or their overall lives. Another smaller group of mothers indicated signs of psychological distress. For mothers, the key factor in these outcomes appeared to be their partner's contribution, or rather lack of it, to family life and the tasks of parenting. The greatest discontent was expressed by mothers who were employed for long hours, that is mothers who effectively did two full-time jobs, but the unhappiness relating to their husband's non-involvement was not confined to employed mothers. These researchers found that women bear the burden of parenting far more than men; some women are both caregivers and breadwinners. Brannen and Moss (1991) have suggested that women's increased involvement in the labour force has not been matched by a corresponding growth in the domestic contribution of fathers. When women are not in the labour force, but are fully employed as mothers, they appear to carry most of the responsibility for parenting and for the domestic chores. O'Brian (1981) suggests that modern man is more nurturing, more responsive and more emotionally involved in his children but Bjornberg (1992) suggests that men are marginalised, redundant and victims of the loss of patriarchal power. In this study, the men have not only lost their patriarchal power, but in most cases they have lost their position as providers. Women have made them redundant and have taken active decisions to live without them. The women in this study have decided to 'go it alone'; many believe that they will make a better job of parenting without the support of the man.

LOOKING FOR SUPPORT AND LIVING ALONE

Kirsty [21] was 23 years old and single. She had three children from three different relationships and was at the time of the study having a relationship with Michael. More than anything, Kirsty wanted Michael to be with her during the birth of her child. She had spent a great deal of time describing her previous childbirth experiences and desperately wanted to have Michael's support in labour, but she said, 'He doesn't like hospitals, he goes all squeamish. He won't come in with me.' I asked if Michael lived with her; she replied, 'On and off, well more or less, he lives with his Mam, he's on and off here really.' She explained further:

> **'Michael did live with me for a bit, but it didn't work out like we wanted to, but we are thinking about it with this one [her current pregnancy]. You know we might make a go of it and start claiming together. People say you get £10 more if you claim together, for the family, the kids and that. The thing is I like it on my own now, he has some meals here but I like being on my own. When the kids have gone to bed, I curl up on the sofa and I have the remote control for the telly. I can wear leggings, drink warm milk, I like the space to myself, no rows, it's just better really, I shall probably carry on like this. My Mam looks out for me, she helps if I am in trouble not him. That's the way it has to be I think.'**

This example illustrates how Kirsty has resolved her situation. The world around her has changed; the collapse of the manufacturing industry has contributed to Michael's unemployment and indirectly to her position. Her partner is not able to support her physically or emotionally, but she feels that by living alone she has regained control over her life and accepts those aspects that she cannot change. For Kirsty, having experienced living in an environment with a restless, insecure man, she believed that she would be better living alone. Initially, the need for respectability seemed to make her believe that a man would provide her and her children with the security they needed; she would, as she said, 'be able to bring my kids up proper'. However, after short stints with men who would return to their 'Mams', go night fishing and seem mentally absent, and who do not offer the support that these women believed they needed, they decided to live alone. For the women in this study who were now having other children with at least a second father, they appear to have taken control over their lives and their situation. The sense of control that these women have leads them to conclude that they have a power over their lives. This power is seen in their control of their finances and in the minutiae of their daily lives.

'PUTTING UP AND PUTTING OFF'

In this section, I first want to describe the life and times of Paul and his ongoing relationship with both Jenny [5] and Sharon [9]. Paul's life style and actions were not unique in the area, but his case was especially interesting. These vignettes illustrate the complexities of relationships that existed in this group of women and how one woman, Jenny, chose to tolerate difficult aspects of her relationship. The following extract is drawn from my field notes.

'One day I went to visit Jenny at her home; I had previously met and spoken with her at the Doctor's surgery. Jenny was 26 years old; she had six previous pregnancies and was the mother of five children. She described herself as cohabiting and had three children from her first marriage, as well as two in her current relationship. Jenny was a warm and sociable person, very willing to talk and share her experiences. Having checked I was nothing to do with Social Security she proceeded to share her views on any subject. She introduced me to Paul, as 'her other half'. He arrived wearing jeans and a vest. Jenny explained that he had just got up (it was midday), as he had been out night fishing. Jenny proceeded, with no prompts, to tell me about her relationship with Paul. Paul wandered in and out, offered me tea and dozed in front of the television. Jenny had been married to Garry for three years, but had now divorced him. The divorce was traumatic and in her opinion of no benefit.' [Field Note]

Jenny [5] said:

'I got no money from him then and no money from him now, it's all a waste of time. That's why I will never marry Paul; it doesn't give you any more security than just living together. We don't live together because of the social; according to them he lives with his mother. But he is the father of these two and the next one. For now I'll just put up with him, perhaps later I'll do something about him. Now I need to have a man around, even if he's not the perfect guy.'

Jenny uses the notion of money to signify something much more complicated. She explains that despite the attractions of a respectable social status, 'married with children', she is better off on her own. She uses money as a symbol of her insecurity in the relationship. Her relationship with Paul was not satisfactory; in her words, 'it's all a bit of a pain really'. She knows things are not right but she *'puts up'* for the sake of the children and to be 'respectable' and she *'puts off'* leaving him at this stage. She would like to be married to Paul but accepts that it is not an available option. She said:

> **'My mother would like me to do the "right" thing. You know be married and that. So would I, but I am not sure it would work anyway. It did not work with Garry. Men have to do their own thing, you know like fishing. The kids need a father, I suppose. I put up with it for them really. I know it's not right, but what is?'**

She then went on to explain that Paul worked on the fairground. They had known each other for many years, and when he was in town, he would look her up and they would meet.

Two days later I visited Sharon [9]; she was aged 16 and single. She explained that her partner was Paul. He had worked on the fairground, manning the stalls. In the past when the fair was in town he would call and see Sharon and they would go out. Paul did not work now, but he was the father of her child born two weeks previously. Sharon explained that the CSA (Child Support Agency) was only interested in Paul if he had a job, and as he was unemployed they would not pursue him. Sharon explained to me how Paul spent a great deal of time on his hobby, night fishing, and was away most of the time. Sharon explained that Paul lived with her 'on and off', but often went back to his mother. Some time later Paul arrived at Sharon's house and let himself in with a key. He nodded to me, offered me tea and sat on the sofa. This Paul was indeed Jenny's other half and had recently fathered two children in the same vicinity. Sharon had no idea that she shared her partner with another woman.

I felt sure that Jenny had some idea about what was going on. There were times in the conversation that she would raise her eyes to the ceiling and say 'night fishing'. These gestures led me to believe that she knew about Paul's life style and was prepared to put up with it. In this example, I have explored the different ways in which different women cope with the difficulties in their relationships. It was clear that Paul's behaviour was unacceptable to me, but Jenny did accept it. I am sure that other people knew about Paul and the position he held in at least two women's lives. In the search for a partner, it appears that Jenny, at least, was prepared to tolerate his life style. Faced with the need to be with a man and be respectable, she was willing to tolerate being with a man who was not loyal to her and who failed to provide for her and her family. The implications of future incestuous relationships between her children and Sharon's children were not considered by either party. She had a very individual way of coping with her relationship with Paul. In her own individual way she had normalised her life, made it acceptable and used her knowledge/power to gain control of her situation. There are no universal accounts of women and their relationships and certainly no universal solutions to their 'problems'.

UNPLANNED PREGNANCIES AND RESTLESS MEN

Sarah [8] was a 15-year-old woman whom I first met in the late stages of her first pregnancy. She lived at home with her mother, her father, her two sisters and their two children. The household was overcrowded and the two elder sisters had been allocated alternative accommodation in the area. They both planned to move out once Sarah's baby was born. Sarah had seen her sister's children growing up and wanted to share in their experience. Sarah wanted children because she believed that she would never be lonely with them and, like many other women in the study, children were essential to enjoy Christmas. She did not plan to become pregnant but misunderstood the advice offered by her GP on the use of the contraceptive pill. She believed that the pill offered protection from pregnancy as soon as she took the first tablet. She became pregnant during the first cycle. She explained that she met the father of her child whilst at work and became pregnant quite quickly after. She said:

'When I told him I was pregnant he was all right at first but then he went like all funny. He has lost the two of us; I've only lost him. Darren [the father] says that he will call to see me if it's a lad, but not if it's a girl. He rang the other day to ask how I was, he could not talk for long, he was in the pub. He likes his beer. I am better off without him; he would only take my money for beer. I like the peace and quiet; I am better off on my own. He thinks he can have the babby on Saturday on his own, but only if it's a boy. He has got another thing coming.

I did think that if I got pregnant he would stop with me, but not for long. I didn't mean to get pregnant, it just happened. He did ask me to get rid of it, but I told him no. I don't believe in it. I didn't get pregnant to keep Darren. It was not about keeping Darren. He has lost nothing. He is probably glad to have escaped from all this.'

I asked Sarah if she thought her life would be any better if she was married or living with a man. She said:

'**No, not really. It depends if he was at work, moneywise it helps. But... If he is on the social he is no good to you. "You know no wage, no use", that's what they say about men.**

At the moment I don't want a man, I couldn't be bothered, they are just a waste of time.'

Thus it appears that in the lives of these women, men are virtually redundant. Not only have men lost their economic power and their patriarchal dominance but also they have lost the value of a close, nurturing and supportive relationship.

Women like Sarah were not interested in the social and political theories that analyse the decline in the interest and respectability of men. The fundamental lesson that most women in this study learned was how to survive best. They looked to their mother for support and quickly learned how to protect themselves. If these disinterested young men were put under a pressure to perpetuate the social image of the perfect father, the night fishing increased and their absence became more dominant. The women learned that it was best to expect little from the men and protect themselves. They found individual and different responses to their situation.

OF SOME VALUE?

One woman, Joanna [22], had been living with her partner for seven years. She was a diabetic and together they had two children and were expecting a third. Trevor, her partner, was unemployed but had had a variety of jobs in the past. They both agreed that working for low wages was counterproductive and that financially they were better off claiming income support and the other housing benefits that were part of the package. For some months, he had been receiving sickness benefit following a back injury. He worked around the house and did odd jobs for other people. Joanna wanted Trevor to stay with her during her labour but she knew it would be her mother or sister. She explained, 'he doesn't like to see me in pain, he's frightened to be honest'. In a more reflective mood and in a subsequent interview Joanna said:

'**Being a parent is really hard work. Three children need a lot of looking after; you need a man there as well. You need some support. Sometimes you get a bit down, you need a break. They play up and it helps to have someone**

**else there. I don't think I could cope if he got work. He'll
not get a job now, not while they are small. We would lose
too much money. We make the most of what we've got
but it's a struggle, it would be worse on my own.**'

Joanna's solution was different. For her, living with Trevor was the right
thing to do. They had resolved their financial difficulties. They were better
off than other women in the study were because Trevor received sickness
benefit as well as housing and other benefits. She weighed up the benefits
and costs and found in favour of living with Trevor. Like the other women,
Joanna used her knowledge of her life, her financial benefits and the
emotional benefits of living with a man and decided she was better off with
Trevor than without him.

SOCIALISING BOYS TO BE BETTER MEN

Claire [24] was older than all the other women in the study; her life
experiences had increased her knowledge and her power. She was angry
and more vociferous in her accounts than other women I met. She came
across as angry, but very much in control. She had clear views and a clear
sense of direction. I interviewed Claire, aged 38, at the GP's surgery; she
had asked to see me. She said that she was very tired, unwell and in the
later stages of her sixth pregnancy. She had three sons by her first marriage
and had suffered a slight stroke in the previous year. She was divorced
and lived with her children. She said that she had heard about me from her
sister and wanted to tell me what she saw as the 'big issues' in the area. She
began by telling me that men were no good and that women were better off
without them. The 'big issues' were drugs, the 'smack heads' that hung
around the streets and the crime. Crime was, in her view, mainly to fund
the kids' drug habits. Most of all she wanted to move herself and her
children away from the area. As she relaxed a little she said:

'**Being a mother is a struggle on your own. Men don't fit
into my life anymore, only my sons. I don't feel that I am
missing out on anything. My ex was a waste of time,
drinking, drugs ... He was a liability. I am having another
baby for me, not for him. Not because I love him or any of
that tosh.**

**I always manage okay, better without him. I am more in
control. He wants to come back but I won't let him. I want
less to do with men. I have brought these up on my own,
it's better. You are your own boss. Men have got attitude,**

they think they can say this, say that, do this, do that. They teach their sons to be rude to women. It's too late for my eight year old, he already thinks that women are stupid, no good, only fit for doing things for men. Cooking cleaning, that sort of thing, they would have women wiping their backsides for them. They don't respect women.

That's what his father taught him, women are dirt to be abused. He taught him that men should go out, sit in the pub and slag off women. On my own I have a chance to bring up boys different to their fathers. On your own you have the chance to bring up your sons how they should be brought up, to respect women.

On your own you can do what you like, go out when you want, stay in when you want. Buy what you want, buy what's best for the kids, not just what he likes. It's too closed in living with a man. Women on their own with kids rely on their own mothers for help. You see it's women, young women, old women grandmothers ... they are the ones who fill the gap and do what men should do. Women just do it.

Most of them are too young to leave their mother. Little boys who can't take the heat. He lived with me and went home to his Mam for tea. Too young to leave his mother, hasn't grown up. Little boys out to play at the pub with their mates, I am better being my own boss. I don't give a shit about what anyone thinks of me. I am not staying with a man just to look right.'

Claire had given up on being respectable. Her anger was directed at a range of people: doctors, midwives, health professionals and men. She was angry and had rationalised her position without a man. She explains that she 'manages okay', that she is better off without him and is explicit about being 'more in control'. She clearly believes that being on her own is better for her and better for her children. She sees her role as a mother in terms of socialising her sons to be better men. She does not see the need to be seen as respectable and is convinced of her ability to survive without a man.

SUMMARY

In this chapter, I have explored the changing and varied nature of the relationships between childbearing women living in poverty and the men in their lives. Set in the context of social deprivation, unemployment, complex relationships and the rapidly changing nature of households and families in the 1990s, I have shown how these women have found many different ways of resolving issues in their relationships. For many women, pregnancy adds physical and psychological pressures and for some women it leads to additional pressures on their relationships with the men in their lives. Such problems are complex; there is not a simple causal relationship between poverty, pregnancy and difficulties in relationships that can be solved by the state and its structures. Simply promoting marriage by offering financial incentives or measures to make divorce more difficult will not solve the problems for women. I have demonstrated how in an ethnographic study such as this, there is no universal problem, no universal account of childbearing women living in poverty and equally no universal solutions to be imposed by academics or the state. Such observations however do not permit the academics nor the state to avoid seeking solutions. The structures put in place to manage the unreliable restless men and ease women's reliance on the state – such as marriage, tax benefits, the work of the CSA – all go some way to alleviate the problems that these women encounter. However, the individual problems and concerns of these women explored in this chapter highlight the gaps that are left by such universal policies. No structure will alleviate all problems, yet by acknowledging this and investigating the individual problems and responses, our understanding of why such structures are failing will improve. It is insufficient for politicians, for example, to attempt to ostracise single mothers by stating that they are merely seeking accommodation. Solutions will not be found by encouraging people to 'shop' benefit fraud. The lack of understanding stems from the confidence that universal structures provide universal solutions. This ethnographic process demonstrates that this is not the case.

Above all this chapter recognises the ways in which individual women balance the need to conform and be respectable with the need to regain control and live alone. In short, individual women find individual solutions to their individual and disparate lives.

In the next chapter, I will focus on other women in the study who also made decisions to stay in relationships. The decision to stay in abusive and violent relationships is more difficult to understand but demonstrates the complexity of relationships and the ways in which individuals seek out individual solutions to their problems.

7

Domestic abuse: different women, different problems and different solutions

INTRODUCTION

Throughout this research, I could not ignore the issue of domestic abuse. It became a key theme and an area where I found even more evidence that there was no universal experience, no universal response and certainly no universal solution to what was clearly a widespread issue. Domestic abuse had obvious physical, psychological and emotional effects on women and on their pregnancies. It became important to uncover the variety of ways in which they adapted to violence and coped with what I felt were difficult and distressing relationships. Some women described how they had been 'knocked about a bit' by their partners; others suffered severe injuries requiring medical attention. Many women told me how they felt that in some way they were responsible for the violence; I learned how some women would avoid contact with me when they had visible bruises or injuries.

It has not been my intention to include all of the extensive and rapidly growing literature in this field. There are many excellent sources of up-to-date and relevant information and advice for midwives (see for example *Midirs*, Midwifery Digest Supplement, 2 September 2002). The purpose of the book is to explore some of the individual ways in which some women experience and choose to deal with domestic abuse. The study draws on the responses and words of individuals in order to examine the very different ways in which women experience domestic abuse.

In this chapter I begin by considering some of the definitions and prevalence of domestic abuse and I briefly review the effects on women's mental and physical health. In the next section I review some of the literature exploring issues of domestic violence and childbirth and in particular focus on the latest *Confidential Enquiry into Maternal Deaths* (HMSO 2001). I try to unravel the issue of who is to blame and consider the so-called triggers of abuse. I introduce 'Dawn's story' [16] and discuss the use of interview data in ethnographic research. I then present an unedited version of Dawn's story.

Much of the medical and nursing literature presented assumes that there is a universal and consistent link between patriarchy and abuse. This is combined with a belief that 'the truth' is out there only waiting to be found. Various theories that attempt to explain and even excuse domestic violence are considered as the researchers in these areas seek to find the 'truth'. The conflicting accounts and theories serve to confirm that there is no one truth and no one reason why some men abuse some women, even during pregnancy. The published research continues to report survey after survey where the researchers try to uncover the incidence of violence, define the victims and offer standard solutions.

I have used Dawn's story to illustrate the unique nature of this violent relationship and the complexities around one woman's efforts to survive in the relationship. The story is useful as it illustrates one woman's struggle to make sense of her life in poverty and her experiences with an abusive partner. Throughout the interview, there is clear evidence of Dawn putting her children first and considering their needs before her own. It also illustrates the pressures around being respectable and 'normal' as Dawn describes her belief that 'any man is better than no man'. Dawn's story is important because it confirms that it is impossible for Dawn, let alone any researcher, to find a simple solution to the problems in her relationship.

In this chapter I also consider 'Emma's story' [25]. Emma minimises the violence and seems resigned and accepting of the violence that is part of her life. She also appears to believe that 'any man is better than no man', even when that man subjects her to physical violence. She believes that her children need a father around. Her story is equally complex; she explains how despite consistent violence she remains 'with' her partner who is the father of her child.

In the next section, I explore some of the reasons why some women in this study decided to stay in abusive relationships. Despite common themes, there was always evidence of individuality and subjectivity. Whilst it was important for many women to be seen as respectable, they presented many different explanations of their own analysis of their positions.

In the final section, I seek to determine the range of tactics that these women used to cope with violence. They became adept at handling complex and different situations in very different ways. They learned to know 'what gets him going' and that to survive they had to avoid 'winding him up'. Therefore, despite the apparent limited options open to the women in the study, they appeared to survive and minimise the assaults on them. They rejected any attempts to work with standard, prescribed, imposed solutions.

DEFINITIONS OF DOMESTIC ABUSE

There is no universally accepted definition of domestic abuse or domestic violence. However, definitions of abuse are very important; they form part of policy statement, action plans and national strategies, and definitions are used to make explicit the philosophy and underpinning beliefs of the group or organisation. Physical violence is clearly only part of the story; emotional, sexual, psychological and financial abuse must be part of any definition. Domestic violence is most commonly described as the systematic abuse, both physical and mental, which takes place in the context of the family structure. The 1993 Home Affairs Select Committee Report on domestic violence defined it as 'any form of physical, sexual or emotional abuse which takes place within the context of a close relationship' (Home Office 1993). The distinction between mental, physical and sexual abuse is also important because it recognises that violence can be far more than a physical assault; it can be bullying, humiliation and degradation. For the woman herself, abuse is abuse, however it is inflicted. In Scotland, the term 'domestic abuse' is the preferred term as this more accurately reflects that violence is only one form of abuse. Domestic abuse also embraces sexual, emotional and even financial abuse. It is generally agreed that whilst men are predominantly the perpetrators and women and children predominantly the victims, domestic abuse can occur in any intimate relationship. Some definitions recognise that domestic abuse is characterised as the misuse of power and the exercising of control by one partner (usually a man) over the other (usually a woman) in an intimate relationship. (For more discussion on this issue see Hunt and Martin 2001.)

THE INCIDENCE

According to the British Medical Association (BMA 1998), Andrews and Brown (1988) and Mooney (1993), at least one in four women will experience domestic violence at some time in their lives, irrespective of their age, social class or ethnicity. These figures are likely to be underestimated because many women will not willingly disclose abuse. Counting and recording the incidence of abuse is equally difficult and the published statistics are fraught with difficulties. However, there is still some convincing evidence that domestic abuse continues to be a major public health issue. This is graphically illustrated in a recent Women's Aid report. On the Women's Aid website it is reported that over 35,000 women called the national helpline in 2000 and in any one day nearly 7,000 women and children are sheltering from violence in refuges in the United Kingdom (Abraham 2000).

In Britain, 25 per cent of all violent assaults are carried out on women by their partners (Lovenduski and Randall 1993) and one in five British murder victims are women murdered by their partner or ex-partner (Smith 1989). In contrast, violence against men by their partners seems to account for just 1 per cent of reported violence, and there is some indication that such violence may be in the form of self-defence (Bakowski *et al.* 1983). As with documented statistics about violence against women, the numbers of men reporting such incidences may be unrepresentative of the actual numbers experiencing such violence. However, even with massive under-reporting of abuse, female violence against men receives a disproportionate amount of media attention and appears to stimulate much more reaction than the infinitely more common abuse against women.

Hence, it is generally agreed that whilst domestic abuse is probably under-reported, between one in three and one in four women are abused by their partners (Radford *et al.* 1998). The literature also suggests that the nature of violence, like the nature of women's responses, varies considerably. The highest reported incidence of domestic violence is amongst those in lower socio-economic groups but women of all classes, ages and ethnic backgrounds experience the crime (Hester *et al.* 1996). Of all the crimes reported to the British Crime Survey 2000, more than 1 in 20 were classified as domestic violence and almost a quarter (23 per cent) of all violent crime is categorised as domestic violence. In 1999, 37 per cent of female homicide victims were killed by present or former partners; this compares with 6 per cent of men (Home Office 2001:76). Women are at greatest risk of homicide at the point of separation or after leaving a violent partner.

In recording and reporting abuse there are other complex issues. It could be argued that a relatively minor incident such as a push or shove might be remembered and reported by an individual, especially if such an action was highly unusual or a one-off incident. For many women the daily grind of physical and emotional abuse may lead them to consider the behaviour 'normal' and as such not worth reporting. Many critics of domestic violence statistics argue that minor injuries are a normal part of complex relationships. Such comments are evidence of the process of 'normalisation'. Discourses define what is normal, in this case 'minor injuries', and consequently what is not normal (violence against women) is then seen as in need of normalisation, or conformity to the norm (Ramazanoğlu 1993). One woman I spoke to said, 'I know he hits me, knocks me about a bit, men do that. It really hurts and makes me scared, I just wish it didn't hurt so much, that's all.'

DOMESTIC ABUSE AND HEALTH

It is widely accepted that violence against women by male partners and ex-partners is a major public health problem. It results in many different types of physical injuries and in a range of mental and physical health problems, some of which can have long-term consequences. It has dire effects on women's mental health and detrimental effects on women and their pregnancies. The Chief Medical Officer highlighted the consequences of domestic abuse in his annual report, *On the State of the Public Health For The Year 1996* (DoH 1997). Exposure of children to domestic violence is known to result in emotional, behavioural and health problems (Humphreys 1993). Stark and Flitcraft (1996) found that almost two thirds of abused children were living in families where the mother was being abused. The effects on mental health are significant: post-traumatic stress disorder, depression, anxiety, lower self-esteem, substance abuse, self-harm and suicide are all reported (Stark and Flitcraft 1996).

Domestic violence is a factor in at least one in four suicide attempts by women (Stark and Flitcraft 1996). The psychological effects of abuse can include low self-esteem, dependence on the perpetrator, hopelessness about ending the violence, and a tendency to minimise or deny the violence (Kirkwood 1993).

DOMESTIC VIOLENCE AND CHILDBIRTH

Domestic violence in pregnancy has an adverse effect on both the woman and her unborn child. At worst it may result in the death of either or both. It is rarely an isolated event and can escalate in severity and frequency during pregnancy (Andrews and Brown 1988). We know that it can lead to recurrent miscarriage, low birth weight, fetal injury, fetal death, stillbirth and maternal deaths (Hunt and Martin 2001:111, Mezey and Bewley 1997a). Domestic violence is also associated with death, severe morbidity, miscarriage, depression and suicide, as well as alcohol and drug abuse. The incidence of domestic violence in pregnancy is unknown (Bewley *et al.* 1997). No one really knows how many miscarriages are direct results of violence and no one can really be sure how often premature labour is caused by violence. In this study, out of 25 women, eight women had had a miscarriage in their pregnancy history. According to Bohn (1990) most studies report a prevalence of abuse in pregnancy of approximately 50 per cent. It is likely that domestic violence is massively under-reported, but it is probably more common than pregnancy-induced hypertension or gestational diabetes (Mezey and Bewley 1997). Both of these conditions are routinely screened for at each antenatal clinic visit.

Most published research suggests that domestic violence may commence or escalate in pregnancy (Mezey 1997). Andrews and Brown's (1988) study of working-class women in Islington reported that 25 per cent had been subjected to violence by their partner. Helton *et al.* (1987), using a questionnaire design, found that of 290 pregnant women attending an antenatal clinic, 23 per cent of women reported violence. In this study 8 per cent reported violence during pregnancy and another 15 per cent disclosed violence prior to pregnancy. Hillard (1985) found that 10.9 per cent of women attending an obstetric and gynaecology clinic reported abuse at some point in the past, and 3.9 per cent reported abuse in their current pregnancy. One in five of these women were still living with the abusive partner.

In the 1994-96 *Confidential Enquiries into Maternal Deaths in the United Kingdom* report (DoH *et al.* 1998), there are reports of six deaths of pregnant women who all were apparently murdered by their husband or partner. The recommendations in the 1997-99 enquiry report, *Why Mothers Die* (DoH *et al.* 2000), are broadly unchanged but all health professionals are strongly encouraged to read the report more fully. The report makes crucial points and sets out the stark reality of the impact of domestic violence on childbearing women. Lewis (2001) points out that 45 (12 per cent) of the 378 women whose deaths were reported to the enquiry had voluntarily reported violence to a health-care professional during their pregnancy. It is believed that this is an underestimate of the true prevalence of domestic violence. There were eight women murdered by partners or close relatives and two others who possibly died as a direct result of violence. Four of these women were living in refuges. In this report 80 per cent of the schoolgirls or young women under the age of 18 whose deaths were considered by the enquiry had suffered violence in the home. The report details the difficulties with communication and how, although some women were offered 'all appropriate support', they were still murdered. Many women reporting violence booked late or were poor attenders at the antenatal clinic yet it was unusual for these women to be actively followed up. The report also draws attention to the inappropriate use of relatives as interpreters. Interpreters are essential in all health-care settings where there is a non-English-speaking population. It is very important for all women to be able to communicate directly with the midwife. Children are not the most suitable interpreters and professional expert and independent translators are crucial. This is a complex area; midwives and other health professionals need expert advice and support as they deal with multifaceted cases. They also need some level of formal training to enable them to support women. The key recommendations in chapter sixteen of this enquiry (Lewis 2001) are worthy of discussion. All health professionals are urged to adopt a non-judgemental and supportive response to women who have experienced physical, psychological or sexual abuse. They are encouraged to provide basic information, and continuing support, whatever decision the woman makes about her future.

The issue of screening childbearing women is still subject to debate (Ramsay *et al.* 2002) but what is clear is that asking questions requires careful preparation, sensitivity, time and a willingness to accept whatever the woman chooses to say and do, or not say and do.

It is interesting and salutary to note that for the first time it has been possible to calculate the social class of women who had a maternal death. The results confirm what has long been expected: women in lower social classes have a higher risk of maternal death. Women from the most deprived circumstances appear to have a 20 times greater risk of dying of direct or indirect causes than women from social classes I and II (RCOG 2001:42). One of the key recommendations of this report states:

'Health professionals who work with disadvantaged clients need to be able to understand a woman's social and cultural background, act as an advocate for women, overcome their own personal and social prejudices and practise in a reflective manner' (2001:45).

It seems that there is still some way to go; providing individualised care is straightforward when the woman shares the midwives' own culture, beliefs and values and has adopted a life style which is easy to support and approve. It is more difficult when the woman appears to be deviant and reluctant to conform, but here we see how in fact it is that woman who is more vulnerable and in greater need of individual care.

WHO IS TO BLAME?

In this study there was some evidence that some midwives and other health professionals believed that domestic violence was somehow the women's fault and that some inadequacy in their nature or action had led to the abuse. The local community midwives were aware that some men were occasionally abusive, but there were no records of domestic violence having occurred during the pregnancy of any woman involved in this study. Yet over half of the sample had experienced domestic violence in the previous year. Many women had been abused during their pregnancy or in the postnatal period. It is not helpful to apportion blame; many women felt guilty and in some way responsible for the abuse. If women do feel responsible they are much less likely to seek to disclose the abuse or seek help in dealing with their difficulties.

TRIGGERS FOR ABUSE

Domestic violence is rarely an isolated event; it can start at any point in a relationship and is likely to increase in frequency and severity over time. The birth of a baby is a major life change; it changes relationships and patterns of life within families and is often a very stressful event in the lives of women. Although childbirth is a normal, expected life experience, it is included in various stress-rating scales, such as Holmes and Rae (1967), as a stressful life event. The changes that pregnancy and childbirth bring are challenging for most women. The physical demands are significant, and the psychological adjustments are considerable; the changes to the social networks within a family require major adjustments. In some circumstances, such changes may be linked to domestic violence.

Stress, however it is defined, is a well-documented trigger of domestic violence, and pregnancy and childbirth are undoubtedly stressful events in the lives of both men and women. Part of the stress undoubtedly comes from the conflict between the unrealistic expectations of parenthood and the demanding reality where the rewards take some time in coming. However, domestic violence is much more than hurting someone physically and psychologically and to explain it away using 'stress' is mistaken. Through violence, the perpetrators exert power and seek to control those whom they assault. Through this control and aggression, vulnerable pregnant women are less able to defend themselves, less able to take evasive action and so more likely to suffer serious adverse effects on themselves and their unborn child. The violence may be physical, sexual, emotional and/or psychological. The abusers or perpetrators of violence are exercising their power and using it to diminish some women's control. When a woman is abused, she loses control; this loss of control is also seen as women being locked into compulsory heterosexual, and therefore respectable, relationships. When a woman is in a relationship with an abusive man, she loses control of her own life and responsibility for her own happiness. In this chapter, I will examine some of the ways in which some women attempt to regain this control. Some women develop tactics that allowed them to acknowledge the abuse, recognise its effects and attempt to change the situation, but all women handle the abuse differently.

SOME WOMEN'S STORIES

In the next section, I will focus on Dawn and on Emma. Dawn's story is important because it illustrates the unique nature of a violent relationship. The complexities of the issues that unfold during the interview serve to reinforce the view that it is impossible to find a simple or common solution. Dawn's story is also interesting in that it provides further evidence of the strong sense of responsibility that some women had for their children. Many of Dawn's decisions were influenced by the needs of her children. Her children's needs were the priority even when her life was extremely difficult.

Dawn [16], a 36-year-old mother of five children, asked to meet me and told me her story. I have presented much of the transcribed interview. This interview is, as Burgess (1980) describes, 'based on a sustained relationship between the informant and the researcher'. The level of detail and the openness and honesty came out of a previous three-hour interview where we talked about many other aspects of her life.

Emma's story, although less detailed, follows on similar lines; this story is included to illustrate the similarities and differences in women's experiences of domestic abuse. It is similar in that both women felt that any man was better than no man. Emma minimises the violence in her life and relationship and appears accepting and resigned to her situation. Dawn has moved on; she is angry and wanting to regain control of her life.

Dawn's story is quite long, but it portrays the complexity of an abusive relationship and some of the pressures on this childbearing woman living in poverty. The controlling nature of abusive men and the cycle of violence described by Walker (1984) are clearly illustrated. There is clear evidence of her putting her children first, the impact of alcohol and drug use on the relationship and the extent of the guilt and fear that dominated that relationship. It also illustrates the belief, expressed by many women, that things would get better, and that change was imminent. It reveals the pressure that Dawn felt was placed on women to stay in an abusive relationship; the pressure to be with a man is marked in a society where single is considered deviant. Dawn said: 'Any man is better than no man.' This, it seems, includes a man who for 20 years has abused her and constrained her.

THE USE OF INTERVIEW DATA

Mayall *et al.* (1999) argue that researching the lives of disadvantaged groups is fraught with issues of power and prejudice; it is crucial that the researcher allows the voices of the researched to be heard. Silverman warns against over-analysis and over-interpretation (1998). In all circumstances, the researcher has to be true to the researched; the data must be reliable, credible, trustworthy and honest. Qualitative research such as this seeks to be close to the data and written from the perspective of the insider. It aims to produce rich, real, deep data. Dawn's story is rich, deep and real. Oakley (1999) argues that, like everything else, research tools have been subjected to the process of social construction. A key part of this social construction has been a 'gendering' of method and methodology whereby 'qualitative' approaches have been aligned with less powerful social groups. She concludes that debates about method are less important than the issue of trustworthiness and selecting the best method for the research question. I believe that had I been male, the interview would have taken a different line. The richness of the data and the credibility of the evidence owe much to the fact that I am a woman. The interview with Dawn clearly demonstrates that in this case the appropriate method was chosen to investigate the lives of childbearing women in poverty.

Atkinson (1995), in his book on the work of haematologists, describes how he uses data extracts to illustrate and develop his arguments. He explains how he does not rely on short snippets and quotes lifted out of the data but he prefers to use a smaller number of *extensive* sequences of data. He argues that he has been struck by the need to preserve the form of the talk and the interaction. In this chapter, it seemed inappropriate to rely only on short quotes. The complexity of the issues and the intensity of the feelings generated by those women who chose to speak with me are best reflected by a long data extract. As I transcribed the interview I added the grammar; I positioned the full stops and commas where I felt appropriate. The result is my interpretation, my perception of the pauses, tone and paragraphs.

DAWN'S STORY

Second follow-up interview.
    Separated, pregnant [due in early July], on state benefits. Living in house owned by a Housing Association.

Left a message at the GP, wants to see me. Note said: SHEILA (for midwife doing research). I've got plenty more to tell you. Come to my house on Friday afternoon.

Sheila: So where would you like to start?

Dawn: Well ... I am thirty-six, pregnant, this is my sixth pregnancy, I was married at 18.

The violence started at least twenty years ago. I met Jim when I was 14. I was very unhappy at home, my parents had split up but I was doing well at school and had lots of ambitions.

From the early days Jim was controlling, he hated me speaking to anyone else and of course I had no other boyfriends.

I had no idea he was violent, I just felt that he loved me and that he wanted to look after me. He used to get angry if I was late or if I did anything without asking him first.

So you just don't see what is happening at all. I did not come from a background where there was any violence at all. My family were ... my father was quite authoritarian but we all had the greatest respect for him. He was a proud man, brought his wage packet home, and gave it to my Mum. She dealt with everything in the house, she had her own friends, and she could do what she liked. She had freedom ... so all this was alien to me but I found myself very confused about that situation.

And um ... I could not understand why he was possessive of my time. I found myself making excuses over time, to my family.

The violence started, not severe violence, but verbal at the

beginning. He would be critical of me, how I dressed, how I spoke, how I looked after the kids.

S: So how did the violence develop ... you said that it started 20 years ago ...

D: Well right from the start, I knew that I was making a mistake then. I was 18, the controlling started straight away. I was afraid, I didn't know how to get out of it. I knew how he would react if I left him because whenever... If ever I hinted that the relationship was not working and I wanted to go he would say that he loved me and could not go on without me, he said he would die ... even at that stage I was frightened ... I knew if I left him how he would react. Whenever I said I wanted out he would say that he loved me so much he could not live without me and would die if I left him. I was frightened ...

S: When you first got married were you both working?

D: Um I was working in a little sweat shop [a factory], he has done bits of casual work, he has never had a full time job. But he controls the money. We were always in debt. Always. We had our own house at one point. Um he was earning quite a bit of money, with what I earned we saved up and put a deposit down on a house ... we had been married about five years, it was all unofficial ... you know his earnings ... anyway we were in debt again very shortly, it was going to be repossessed. We managed to sell it just in time.

That was the first time I left him. I realised what was happening, he spent so much money. I went back to my family. They realised that things weren't right, you know, as they should be.

S: I know this is really hard for you, I am really sorry about what has happened to you. It has been difficult for you haven't you ...

[Pause]

S: When did the physical violence start? It sounds as if there was emotional abuse from a very early stage.

D: I can trust you I like talking to you. When did it start um? I can't really put my finger on it... um well yes I can, it was when I was first pregnant. He became physically violent he hurt me badly. I had bruises and cuts most of the time. Once he burnt my arm with a cigarette.

He was always sorry, sorry that he hit me or sorry that he shouted. Then he would turn it around and make out it was my fault. He would say 'If only you hadn't said that ... or if only you hadn't done that.'

I was really worried when he hit me when I was pregnant, I used to cry, sob in bed on my own. I hated it, hated the pain and I hated feeling insulted.

S: Was there any sexual violence? Were you forced to have sex against your will?

D: No, if anything he would withhold it, withhold any kind of affection at all if he was upset with me. It was physical violence, head, tummy, always and bruises.

[Pause/tea]

S: Is there any pattern in the violence that you can see?

D: Yes, there is a pattern, there is the build up, the row,. I could sense it, you know if you say the wrong thing. It was not always when he had a drink, it was most common the morning after when he was, he got a hang over. He ... I would be getting the kids ready for school, doing what you have to do in the morning and he would ... not get up and um ... He would remember something from the night before, some flirting or something, then the arguments would start usually. Um ... I sensed it, he became more tense, and then there would be the explosion. It could just be ... an hour or all night long. He would keep me up all night long. It did not bother him because he could sleep all day, but I had to get up for the kids. And so quite often I was very very, very stressed and very tired, worn out. But um ... I was crying out for help but I didn't know where to turn.

I could not tell my parents ... There are a couple of reasons ... because I did not want them to be hurt, and I was so ashamed that I had put up with it. People assume that if this is happening why doesn't she just leave. But there were so many reasons why I didn't just leave then. But I did, I left many times, I went to my family. It was the same ... the tension, the big explosion [That's when he hit you? Yes.]. Then he would be really sorry.

S: So he was afraid that you were going to leave him?

D: Yes, yes. The first time I went to my sister, to her family, but. She put me up. And um ... I told her what had been going on. They really knew. He would not have anything to do with my family, socially or anything. It was the kids really, they always came first in my mind. Everything I thought of I thought of the kids first. When I was afraid of him, it was fear of... well fear for the kids all the time.

S: You said that it started in your first pregnancy, has it been the same in the others?

D: Yes, I have left him lots of times.

S: What made you come back?

D: Well um a number of reasons. First I left him um after I went to my family. He wrote me long love letters full of remorse, please give me another chance ... I'll never do it again. You know. And the kids of course, always the kids ...

I felt that I owed him another chance ... so I went back. It did work at first; he treated me like a queen ... We would go through this honeymoon period, where you know; we pretended we were in love again. In his way, he was never a good father and husband, he never provided for us, but he improved. Slowly it would take on the same pattern again. I think I thought that any man was better than no man.

S: When you say he improved, in what ways did he improve?

D: Um he allowed me that bit more freedom that I wanted, wasn't so demanding of me around the house. Um and tried in his way to help a bit. I would come back with things on my terms, you know 'you have got to do more around the house ... you have got to get some work'. He had a drug problem and that's where all his money went.

S: What sort of drugs?

D: Cannabis, you know, very large amounts. It was sort of continuous and drink you know. [Pause]

S: When you decided to leave him ...

D: I want to tell you about when I went to hostels.

S: Okay, thanks.

D: I took the children with me. My parents washed their hands of me because I kept going back ... and so I felt very much on my own. The first time I left him and went somewhere else, I rang Women's Aid and went into a home for battered wives. It was a safe house. It was awful.

S: Why was it awful?

D: Everything about it was awful ... it was overcrowded; there were loads of kids. The kids there had behaviour problems, I found my children were bullied. The whole atmosphere was, was ...

I had enough of my own problems, I could not cope with everyone else's as well. I could not cope, I was worried about the effect it was having on my own children ... if you don't put them first you've lost it really, haven't you?

I thought if only he would change and do what he said he would do, then that would be best for the children. He would use the children as well. He would make them feel responsible for getting us back together. He would make them ... he said, 'you want mummy and daddy to get back together don't you?' (This was when he had them on his own.) 'Tell mummy you don't want to change school.'

So they did, and I would feel guilty. Incredibly guilty, the kids are important, so I would go back. Thinking ... well it hasn't all been a waste of time, because now I am going back on my terms. I think he uses the kids, well he uses my feelings about them he knows that they come first all the time, I'm putty really, kids first me next.

S: How often do think that has happened, the cycle you have just described?

D: Many times. Probably once or twice a year. I have been close to a nervous break down many times. I just could not cope.

S: What sort of injuries have you had?

D: Well I had a broken arm, a fractured skull. A damaged kidney, I was passing blood. I lost two teeth once, these are false front teeth. I try not to go to hospital with anything, he would not let me. I suppose it was never that serious. It was mostly bruising around the neck, black eyes, just bruises I suppose.

S: So what is happening now then?

D: The last time I left him ... his drinking was worse, he could not stop drinking, but he stopped going out and was drinking in the house. He wanted my time and demanded my time. I had to sit with him and talk to him; I could not do anything of my own. He was very demanding and I could not cope with that. It became unbearable, his drinking was so bad, and he could barely stand. He just ... so pathetic. I could not live with him in the same way anymore. I didn't ... I just didn't feel the same towards him anymore. I don't want to work at it anymore. I work ... It's just ...

[Pause]

S: Has he got a job?

D: He does fiddles and things. He does foreigners. He could do proper work, you know carpentry, and he made

that table. But ... but he won't carry on. He won't apply himself regularly, it's so frustrating. He would work and then not go in ... if he had too much to drink he would not go in. People don't put up with that, so he never managed to stay anywhere. It was a shame really.

S: The decision to separate has taken a long time.

D: Yes, no well I always knew that I could not spend the rest of my life with him. I ... deep down I always knew that I would have to leave him ... but it would have to be the right time.

The right time never seemed to come it was always the children. I was always pregnant. Still am ... but now it's different.

All of my children were conceived during one of these 'honeymoon' periods ... when we got back together. So each time there was another child there, so it was that much more harder to make the break ... More difficult to leave.

But each time I have got much stronger. In some ways I thank him because he has made me very strong in some ways. I could not have gone through getting into this house if I hadn't have had some sense of justice for myself. If I had not been through all this ...

[Pause, tea, children and other interruptions]

S: So what is the situation now?

D: Well I am pregnant, you can see that! The baby is due in about three months. I left him twelve months ago. The drinking became unbearable, he went to prison ... he was done for drink driving, and it was the second time. He was taken from the court to prison. I thought this was meant to be; this is just what he needed. I saw it as a God send, it will dry him out sort him out. He will come out of prison and not have a drinking problem. It was a terrible shock as well. I wrote to him and visited him and said this is positive, it's a chance to get off the drink, he kept telling me he wanted to stop. He agreed with me, he knew he had got a problem.

But when he came out, he said I have got to celebrate, got to go out. He went out the first night with his friends, not me, he was blazing drunk, and I got pregnant. It was not what we planned.

From then on every night he got drunk. Not in the day. Just at night. I was too tired to cajole him I just ignored him. He was more possessive. He was just the same. More possessive than ever.

Then one evening ... like a fool. The straw that broke the camel's back. One evening ... Every night he used to get me to fetch his beer for him. I said no, you promised me that you would stop; I'm not going to get it tonight. You promised me.

[Pause]

I was taking my son to a friend that night; I decided to call in and see my sister. At that time I only saw my sister once a week because of his possessiveness. I only stayed half an hour and when I came back the office had just closed and he was sitting there waiting for me. He had been phoning around everybody for me. He phoned my mum, my other sister, all because I was half an hour later than I said I had been. He became violent that night. He was torturing me that night. He said he was worried, he said 'I thought you might have had a car accident', making out it was just concern and my fault. I said 'now you know it wasn't an accident and I am okay why don't you let it drop?' He kept saying 'why didn't you phone me'. He kept me awake all night, tormenting me, I was so distraught; I was in such an emotional state I made my mind up there and then.

I said I can't take any more it doesn't matter what happens now, I knew that I couldn't take any more. I had been thinking about doing it for ages, I had phoned up Women's Aid and Focus. They were a new charity in the area, I heard that they had a domestic violence unit, I had spoken to them, and they met me at the hospital one day. It was a new scheme, they were getting it ready. It was always in the back of my mind. And um ... I went to the phone box; I could not use the phone in the house. He was asleep, but he might come down. I rang then left, I was only in jeans and t-shirt, and some clothes for the kids. I had to go somewhere there and then.

I left and lived in the safe house for three years, I could not have done it without the Focus. They had a youth worker or something and she took the kids to school every day. I did not want them to change schools again. They had had enough, enough. The older children have been so disrupted by having to change schools all the time, every day they were messed about. The younger ones were happy where they were and so this worker took them to school every day.

A neighbour would pick them up. He stayed at this house thinking that I would come back, thinking it was just another warning. But it wasn't this time; I am getting too old for this ... I've got to do something permanently. But he still has not accepted it. Even now. I have been to see a solicitor and started the divorce.

S: How did you get your house back?

D: He agreed ... um in fact he decorated it and making it ... you know doing all the things that he said he would do. All the things he should have been doing ... he was getting the house all nice for me for when I come back. He kept writing me all these love letters, telling me to come back. That's how I got pregnant this time.

But I said I want you to move out of the house, let me have the house for the kids.

So he has got himself a horrible little bed-sit flat and moved out. He only got that because he thinks it's just for now. But I've stuck to my guns. I still have had tremendous problems with the kids.

S: Do they want their Dad back?

D: No, they don't want him back, they see that ... um their loyalties are so torn ... they see Mum coping very well but Dad is so ... he's got such a pathetic ... they feel desperately sorry for him. He keeps feeding them with stuff ... Mum has destroyed this family. She has really destroyed this family. They are coming around slowly, to my way of seeing things. But initially, my sixteen year old lad ... I can't take this any more. Let's leave him again. He can't bear to see him hitting me.

When I say he was hitting me, he was never as bad as he used to be. Years ago. He was still violent recently, but my son encouraged me. He was like my best friend. He was encouraging me; he said he needs teaching a lesson. About time Mum. But at weekends he sees his Dad and he comes back confused.

He says: 'you conned me Mum. You told me you were only

teaching him a lesson ... you didn't say you were doing this for good ...' I think he felt betrayed. He wanted it all to be all right I suppose.

He has had a very hard time; he's lost his school. He left school, he did very poorly in his exams, it's all tragic really.

S: Do you think that your relationship with Jim has ended now?

D: Yes, I have started the divorce. It has ended but he is still controlling me. He comes every Sunday for his dinner; he comes to see the children. His flat is so poxy and horrible depressing. He is drinking more than ever now and threatening to throw himself out of his thirteenth floor window, when he is depressed.

I still feel, in some ways, responsible for his emotions. Even now. ... But when I see a pathetic figure and he is your kids' father ... you want the best for them but just give me my freedom please. It's so difficult because the children want to see him and ... I find myself the only time we all get together ...

It has ended but is difficult. Every time he sees the children he is questioning them, where am I going? He searches the house for telephone numbers; he wants to put this fellow off. He has succeeded he's gone now.

He is still not accepting it, he rings he writes. I have made a stand with this. I've got to stand up to him; he is the kids' father and nothing else.

I'd like to emigrate and start again. But I've got a criminal record. You know for the thieving. But I am going to college have a fresh start. I am a fighter; I have friends who believe in me.

And that's that you can go now.

Although this is a long extract, it seemed right and fair to Dawn to present her words without the usual cleaning of the data. Aspects of her story were typical of many women in the study and reveal the complexity of living with domestic violence.

A cycle of violence has been well described in the literature. Walker (1979) describes a gradual build-up of tension, followed by an explosion of violence and then a period of relative calm. The women in this study report that not all domestic violence reflects this pattern and as violence progresses the periods of calm become fewer and there is less evidence of contrition. Some women felt that they precipitated violence or that their actions, simple acts or omissions could trigger an assault. Dobash and Dobash (1977) believe that domestic violence results from real or perceived challenges to the man's position, authority or control over the woman. Browne (1987) reports that many men who batter find the threat of abandonment or rejection by their partner almost unbearable and it may be their extreme neediness that psychologically ties the women to them. Alcohol is an important background factor as well as being a causal or a precipitating factor in violence (Gayford 1978).

All this seemed evident in the story of Dawn, but what became clear is that the causes and effects of violence were often varied and complex. In the same way that she describes her angry and indignant son returning confused, it is impossible for Dawn or researchers to find a concise solution. Dawn finally concluded that it was best to leave. Radical feminism would suggest that the decision to leave should have been made 20 years ago. The fact that Dawn did not leave would be put down to the powerful effect of patriarchy, and if more hostels were available, all would have been well. Dawn, however, cannot identify the true facts as to why she stayed. The interview demonstrates evidence that there is a great responsibility for her children as well as the need to be seen as respectable. How much of this was a response to the middle-class woman sat before her cannot be known. No universal patterns and responses can be drawn from the story of Dawn; what becomes abundantly clear, however, is that the stories such as this are often intricate, complex, multifactorial and beyond simple theorising by either Dawn or the researcher.

EMMA'S STORY

Emma [25] was 15, single and had lived in various addresses. She was pregnant with her second child when I met her. Her first child, born when Emma was 13, had been adopted. She had been abused as a child by her father and by her stepfather. She had spent a brief period of time in care. Since her current pregnancy had been confirmed, she lived with her mother in their council house. Her sister Maria and her child also lived in the same house. She shared a bedroom with Maria and her two-year-old niece Sophie. Her partner, Geoff, lived with her 'on and off'.

She offered to tell me her story not long after I began the research. I had met her at the Friday clinic and had enjoyed a number of chats and discussions with both Emma and her mother. I said very little during the interview. Her mother wanted to stay for the interview but Emma had decided that she wanted to be alone. She told me that she had known Geoff since her school days and that he was her partner and father of her child. The interview was very informal; it was tape-recorded but frequently interrupted by Maria, Sophie and occasionally Emma's mother. I decided to listen and ask questions only when the conversation slowed or paused, which was not very often.

Sheila: Tell me something about your background and life.

Emma: That will be fun, how long have you got. I was born in Walsall and lived with my Mum and Dad until I was about eight I think. My real Dad was a bit mad really, he worked in the leather factory but he and my Mum split up. After you know ...

Anyway Mum married Ed, he is my stepdad. I didn't like him much, so after I got pregnant I went into care for a bit. I went back to school after the baby; I was too young to cope really. You know, it was all too much. I didn't mind the adoption; it was a relief really. I went back to school and lived in the home. I wanted foster parents but that never happened. Anyway I met Geoff when I went back to school, I had always known him and well we sort of got together then. He hit me on the first date, I said something he didn't like and he hit me across the face. I had my first black eye from him at fifteen. It was just like my stepfather in a way. Anyway he was sorry after and said it was a mistake. He was leaving school and had got a job in the butchers. I was leaving too and we thought we could get a flat together. That didn't work out, we couldn't get the deposit and so after I got pregnant Mum said I could move in. Not Geoff but he lives with me on and off.

S: What do you mean by 'living with me on and off'?

E: Well I keep meaning to finish with him. But he comes around, brings some chips and then you know before I know it we are sort of back together again. I think I will be better on my own but perhaps when the baby comes it will be better with a Dad even one who knocks me about a bit.

He can't help it really, it's just that he gets jealous, he hates the hospital you know. He thinks they are sort of interfering with me. He said 'like it's private, it is not for no doctor to go snooping around'. He doesn't mind the midwives so much but he hates the hospital.

S: What do you mean when you say 'he can't help it'?

E: Well he knocks me about; he loses his temper, gets cross and then thumps me. That's when I left the last time. I had a black eye and some bruises on my thighs. He kicked me with his army boots on. I cried but he said it was my fault, I had irritated him.

He said that I was going on about a pram and money and that he had had enough of it. He is always sorry after, he brings me chips and says it will be okay when the baby is born.

It's being going on for ages really, well I met him when we were in school last year. He was jealous then, he didn't like the other guys 'gawping' at me. He did not want to stay in school at all, he wanted to work with his Dad in the factory but there are no jobs at the moment. He will be better when he gets a job. The butcher's shop didn't really work out.

My real Dad was a bastard really, he was always groping and you know, 'our little secret'. My Mum never knew about it, but I think she guessed, anyway she left him and married Edward. My stepdad was just as bad really, he thought I was his property and he could help himself.

He has gone now, well most of the time. He says it's too noisy with Sophie and it will be worse with a new baby.

So Geoff turns up gets cross and frustrated and then loses his rag. That's just the way it is I suppose. I don't finish with him cos we ain't really started. He will be okay when the baby's born.

I sometimes get upset and angry, he really hurts me when he hits me, but I know it will get better. I am better off with him than just with my Mum and sister I suppose.

S: Does Geoff give you any money?

E: No, you must be joking. He hasn't got any anyway. He says if he gives me money it's like paying for sex and I will be a prostitute, so no, no money. I sometimes think I am you know a slag. If we, you know, well it sort of calms him down and then he doesn't get so worked up and cross. Last week he hit me with a table light, I had stitches at the surgery, you know just strips, and it was not too bad. The midwife checked the baby's heart beat while I was there so that's okay. I know that he shouldn't do it, I asked him not to but he can't help it really. He will be a good Dad. He bought a teddy last week from the market. It will get better once the baby's born, I am sure about that. All men do it a bit don't they? My Dad and my stepdad both knocked my Mum about.

S: Have you told anyone at the hospital or the surgery that you are knocked about?

E: No, no one has ever asked. Even when I had the stitches no one said anything. It's up to me really. I think it will get better. I don't know that it's the hospital's

business, well as long as the baby is okay, I suppose that's what matters. What can they do anyway?

S: Thanks Emma.

This interview is interesting as it illustrates Emma's willingness to accept the situation. She believes that 'any man is better than no man' and that a baby needs a father even if that father abuses the child's mother. We see that Geoff suffers from jealousy, has a bad temper and lacks the means to support his partner and child. In Emma we see optimism and a belief that it will get better after the baby is born. She appears to have little faith in the health service's ability to resolve the issue. She does not see the abuse as a problem, providing the baby is all right.

WHY DO WOMEN STAY IN ABUSIVE RELATIONSHIPS?

It was tempting to summarise women's accounts of their relationships and develop lists of actions and explanations. However, I found that by careful analysis of the interview transcripts there was evidence of both individuality and subjectivity. There were similarities in the accounts and some common themes. There was evidence that many women put the needs of their children first. There was also a need to be seen as respectable and being respectable meant being with a man and not living alone.

In the next section I have tried to uncover some of the reasons why women stayed in abusive relationships. The reasons were as varied and different as the women themselves, but the analysis is useful in exposing the variety and complexity of the decisions.

Mel [1] believed that the abuse could be explained as a 'bad patch'. She said:

'Before I divorced him he used to knock me about every Friday night. It was always the same pattern, he would get drunk, he would blame me that there was no money left and then start throwing things at me. I would hide in the back room, but there is no place to hide really. I always thought it was just a bad patch. It didn't make any difference being pregnant. I thought we could get through it, it was worse if the kids were ill or playing up.'

Sally [7] was always afraid that one day her partner's temper might result in the death or injury of either herself or her children. She explained during one interview that the fear that she might be killed was overwhelming, so that was why she stayed. Her mother, present during the interview, constantly interrupted, saying 'Why don't you leave him?'

Sally said:

'It was always the same. He threatened to kill me. Once he explained how easy it would be to kill a woman. He would stand there holding a hammer. He said he would kill me and the kids and then himself. I am scared to death, there is no phone in this house and the one in the street has been vandalised. When he gets in a temper there is no knowing what he might do. After he has calmed down it's okay.'

Claire [24], who was divorced, explained that she had been abused by her husband for many years but always believed that if she changed her behaviour in some way the abuse would stop. She felt that she should stay in the marriage for the sake of her children and because her mother had put pressure on her to avoid the stigma of divorce. Her reasons were embedded in the need to be seen as respectable and the need to conform to her mother's religious beliefs. She said:

'I knew that I would leave him in the end but children need a father and my mother was a Roman Catholic and always felt divorce was a sin. I felt there was always a chance that I could change him. If I were a better wife, he would stop the violence. In the end you just sort of carry on. You convince yourself it's not that bad. You sort of believe it will get better, I used to think that being pregnant would help me, but it never did.'

Gaynor [18] described herself as single; she was 16 years of age and her partner lived with her 'on and off'. Their relationship had lasted some three years. Gaynor was very reluctant to speak about the violence at first but eventually confided in me. The violence had started when she and her partner were both still in school. She had had previous pregnancies that ended in miscarriage and had come to accept violence as part of a relationship with a man. She explained that her mother knew about the violence and had previously confronted her boyfriend at his parents' home. Gaynor believed that violence was a normal part of adult life; she had seen her own mother abused and accepted it was something that men did. Gaynor said:

'I was always knocked about, even when we were in school. He was always sorry. He got frustrated and stressed and then would hit me. At first it was just a slap

or a push but later he would thump me with his fist. I had a black eye last week, that's why I didn't go to antenatal. He goes home to his Mum now he still gets angry. That's men for you.'

Finally Rachel [2] explained why she stayed. Rachel was 22 years old and lived with her boyfriend Craig.

'There is nowhere to go really. It's hard enough to find a place to live without looking for somewhere else. I went to a hostel once but it was terrible so I came home. My mother says I should leave him, I probably will when I am older, but now I am just too tired, what with being pregnant and that. Some say men grow out of it. They settle down and stop the aggression. Perhaps he will. He's always sorry.'

These extracts serve to illustrate the diversity and complexity of both women's lives and the process of rationalising their situation. My research with this group of women has enabled me to suggest some of the reasons why some of these women acted in the way that that they did. Some women believed that the relationship was going through a 'bad patch' and that eventually it would improve. Some women had separated on a temporary basis as their partner had returned to his mother's house. Some believed that violence was an unusual response to a difficult time and they believed that things would soon change for the better. Some were afraid that their partner would carry out his threat to kill her if she left but most women had no extra money at all and to go anywhere would require a bus or taxi fare. One woman described how she stood in the garden, determined to leave, and realised that she had no money at all and nowhere to go. She did not have a telephone and could not ring Women's Aid or any other voluntary organisation. For some women, their children were the reason for staying with abusive men. Some believed that their children needed a father, even an abusive one, and so they stayed. Some women described pressure from their family to stay. One grandmother told me that every man had a right 'to correct' his wife, and that her daughter probably deserved the beating. Most women in this study were convinced that they were responsible for the violence. This premise led them to believe that they could change their behaviour and thus prevent further violence. Some women said that until I had asked them about domestic violence they had not considered it unusual and definitely not a crime. To suggest leaving the relationship was unthinkable as they were unaware there was a problem. This is an obvious contradiction and illustrates the ways in which some women had normalised violence in their lives. Finally, some felt that they were just too tired to do anything about it. To leave a violent relationship would take a great deal of energy and most women led me to believe that they were too exhausted coping with poverty, debt, small children and ill health to do anything about it.

It is not possible to be absolutely sure why some women stay in abusive relationships and why some leave. Some women offered a few explanations: their explanations were partial and limited by the nature of the relationship they had with me. In this research I tried to understand something of the complexities of individual lives so that we might begin to know a little more.

As previously noted, of the 25 women who contributed to this study, 14 had experienced domestic violence in the previous year; all of these women had been physically and psychologically abused during their pregnancies. Some of the injuries were severe and seemed to require medical intervention. However, as can be seen by Dawn's story, the usual practice was to stay in until the bruises had disappeared. Of this group of 14, two women were married, one described herself as cohabiting, five were divorced and six described themselves as single. Those who were single were abused by the men they referred to as their partner. The option of leaving the relationship was not open to them as they theoretically lived alone. The men they described as their partner would live with them 'on and off' and it was during the periods when they lived together that the violence took place. Some women who described themselves as single might be better described as cohabiting but the rules on benefit payments encouraged them to stay single. The women in this study had very complex and very diverse lives.

TACTICS TO COPE WITH DOMESTIC ABUSE

During the extensive interviews with women who had been abused it was possible to determine the tactics they used to cope with violence. This is what the women said:

- 'Never have a go at him on Friday night, especially if he's had a drink.' Emma [25]

- 'Don't say "no job no use" when he can hear you.' Rachel [2]

- 'Always be available, you know, have sex when he fancies it.' Barbara [10]

- 'It's the children who get to him. You have to keep them out of the way if he's tired and that.' Emma [25]

- 'He hates my mother being around, he can't stand it if I'm on the phone to her or if I haven't got the tea in time. That's when he really gets wild.' Sally [7]

- 'Never say you will leave him, it just makes him scared and then he lashes out.' Rachel [2]

- 'Don't have a go at his mother, that's red rag to a bull.' Barbara [10]

And Claire [24]:

'You can handle the abuse, it's not good but you can survive. Just know what ts him going I suppose. Never have a go at his mother, or say you will leave him. Don't wind him up where he can get something to throw at you. It's just common sense really. To survive don't wind him up.

It seemed to me that these childbearing women living in poverty appeared to have very limited options; at best they could hope that the perpetrator of the violence would wander out of their relationship and give them a chance for some peace and quiet. They were severely limited by the lack of money and by a lack of material possessions such as telephones in their homes, a car, even a suitcase to pack to escape. They were committed to their children and would not consider leaving them with their partner in order to escape abuse. Many of these women believed that domestic violence was their lot in life and they had to do only the best they could to minimise the harm. It is also important to consider that the women could have been exaggerating their position; they could have been sharing their stories to get sympathy, attention and understanding. One thing was certain: the fact that they were all very different and did not want anyone imposing common solutions or prescribing a course of action. The issue of professional control is taken up in the next chapter.

SUMMARY

This chapter has drawn on some of the vast literature from a range of disciplines, in medicine, nursing, social work and sociology. I have tried to illustrate the desire these disciplines sometimes have to define, theorise, measure and solve the 'problem' of domestic violence. The research presented here illustrates the unique nature of women's violent relationships and suggests that whilst many women seek to be seen as respectable and frequently put their children's needs above their own, their responses are as varied and different as the women themselves. I have explored women's individual explanations and analysis of their own positions and considered the variety of ways in which they cope with violence. In conclusion, I met with very different women. They were in different age groups, at different stages of their childbearing career, of different marital status, of different religious faiths; they lived in different types of homes and in different family groups. The only common factors were that they were white, heterosexual, pregnant and living in poverty. They were different women with very different solutions to a common problem.

8

'All I want is a bit of respect': pregnancy, poverty and the health professional

INTRODUCTION

This chapter focuses on some women's views of midwives and other health professionals. During the research, it became clear that some women felt strongly that the care they received was dictated by their assumed status, dictated by the area in which they lived, and therefore their social class. Many women felt that midwives and others made judgements about them, their skills as parents and their social worth. These judgements dictated their responses to the women and coloured the nature of their care. Often women strove to be seen as respectable in an effort to counter the negative effects of their social position. In this chapter, I begin by briefly exploring the concept of social class and reiterating the current methods of measuring social class. I then discuss the reasons why midwives and others appear to place such emphasis on what they believe to be the social class position of individual women. All theories of social class rely on the notion of social grouping which tends to assume that all are the same. Midwives have been indoctrinated into this belief from their first days in training. Of course those in social class IV are at greater risk of most things; the evidence, some of which is presented in this chapter, is clear. However, this is a dangerous assumption and as such is the root of many problems in the delivery of care. There is a tendency to assume that all women in class IV are vulnerable, at risk, poor attenders for health care and unlikely to breast-feed their babies.

In the next section, I pose the question, 'Does poverty matter?' I briefly explore the use of the concept of social class in defining and measuring inequalities in health and begin to consider the impact these inequalities might have both on midwives who give care to the women and on the women themselves. The link between poverty and poor health is well established and determines the structured response of the state to what is perceived as a structural issue. Although the health inequalities discourse is firmly based on a structured understanding of poverty and health interventions, its findings and theories have proved robust and useful in targeting health-care provision. These theories cannot be ignored nor swept away by poststructural theorising, which emphasises the individual. The danger, however, is in how midwives and others use and misuse these theories and evidence. The concept of social class and the inequalities in health discourse can be used or abused by some health professionals to the detriment of childbearing women perceived to be and defined as poor (perceived and defined by structuralists, health professionals and others). There is clear evidence that Britain has marked social divisions and inequalities in health. I draw on the work of Wilkinson (1996) to suggest that individuals tolerate social injustice and inequality as if an individual's position in society is a reflection of their innate worth. In this study, and according to some women, some midwives appeared to value them only in relation to their position in society, i.e. in the lowest social class. I explore the theories that attempt to explain the links between social factors and adverse pregnancy outcomes to illustrate the nature and sources of knowledge that is available to midwives and others and which in turn informs their practice.

I present these arguments to explain why some midwives might feel that they are superior to childbearing women in poverty, why they feel that they are more knowledgeable than the women are, and why they may become disenchanted with them. I try to explain why they may consider the women deviant and non-compliant. In the next section, I consider the research evidence that demonstrates that women on state benefits may not be able to afford a healthy diet. The evidence in the scientific published literature is confirmed by this study; the variety and complexities of managing on a low income are explored earlier in chapter four. I conclude this section by confirming that poverty does indeed matter. Not only does it have an adverse effect on the physical and mental health of women, but also it affects the attitudes of some midwives towards some women.

In the next section, I consider certain aspects of the relationships between some women and some health professionals. I explore how some midwives, and others, use and abuse their power and knowledge in their dealings with women. I found that some of the women had better relationships with community midwives than hospital midwives but also evidence that many midwives based their care on assumptions about women's social class and position.

I then briefly explore the attitudes of some midwives towards some of the women who contributed to the study. I consider their beliefs and opinions that some women are poor simply because of their 'inappropriate' life styles. I discuss how some midwives see women living in poverty as uniformly feckless, irresponsible and inadequate and the assumptions that they make about their life styles and spending decisions. I then attempt to explain why midwives perpetuate structures and stereotypes as a means of control and to exert their superiority and power.

The chapter concludes by reiterating the fact that poverty does indeed matter. Not only does poverty have a detrimental effect on some women's mental and physical health, it appears to dictate and inform the quality of care that some women receive from some midwives.

CLASS AND SOCIAL CLASSIFICATION: HELP OR HINDRANCE?

This section explores the literature and arguments that surround the concept of social class. The debates around the relevance of class flourish in both the sociological and medical literature but it is important first to consider why the concept is pertinent in a study of this nature. The research is about childbearing women living in poverty; this chapter focuses on midwives as health professionals and it examines the ways in which the care they offer to women is influenced by their values and beliefs relating to social class. Midwives are a part of the medical profession and are acutely aware of the importance attached to class. As midwives, they are conscious of the arguments and the published literature that make explicit the link between poverty and ill health. These arguments are explored later in this chapter. Such beliefs, knowledge and attitudes are deeply entrenched in the minds of most midwives; this inevitably leads to the views that differences in health are mainly due to differences in class and corresponding life styles. The descriptions of class, with which most midwives are familiar, also carry with them assumptions about life style that may or may not be accurate. Whilst it is clear that patterns of behaviour cannot be assumed to be simply based on class, for midwives, this is often a difficult path to tread. They, like the medical profession, are acutely aware that differences in health are frequently considered as the direct result of differences in class and life style, and there is an assumption that individual social class groups share a common life style. There is also an assumption that those in social class I will share the same healthy life style whilst those in class V will all smoke and eat an unhealthy diet etc. This leads to a belief that poverty is not only associated with a poor life style but that it is life style that leads to greater ill health and earlier death. It is worth noting the belief that ill health also leads to poverty but this is a separate issue. The middle classes, en masse, are thought to eat more healthily, live in better homes, seek medical advice and intervention more readily, respond more willingly to health education messages and are generally considered to be more compliant and obedient. The poor, on the other hand, are thought to be a burden; they are irresponsible, feckless and incompetent and die at an earlier age. They represent a drain on the country's resources and a drain on the midwife's time and energies. Midwives are inculcated into the view that the poor are responsible for their ill health and earlier death and it is the life style of these groups rather than their income which is chiefly responsible. These opinions are derived from the lectures that health professionals receive and from the very culture of the hospital environment. It is these beliefs that allow midwives and others to impose their 'justified' sense of superiority on the poor, the unmarried, those from ethnic minorities and other deviants. The professions have a superiority based on their knowledge. They have a lack of respect for those in a lower position or with a lower status. This then justifies their position and action in treating them in a different way. This begins to explain why some midwives act and respond in the way they do and why it now becomes necessary to explore the concept of class.

Peter Townsend, concluding his book on *Poverty in the UK* (1979), states: 'the theoretical approach developed in this book is one rooted in class relations'. He sees class as a major factor determining the production, distribution and redistribution of resources. He also believes poverty is related to the cultural patterns of society, the life styles that govern 'the expectations attaching to membership of society' (1979:924). In 1993, in tune with many others, Townsend wrote, 'social layers in Britain have been partly reconstituted, more deeply etched and more widely spaced' (1993:92). As this study has revealed, inequalities exist between rich and poor, between women and men. Such divisions are associated with differences in educational opportunities, leisure activities, health prospects, income potential and the power to influence events in society. The stratification is an important starting point for analysing behaviour, and in industrial societies, class is just one of the many strata used to differentiate between people. Social class forms an important theoretical concept, and most commentators accept its existence and significance. As a concept, however, it is extremely difficult to 'operationalise' or use in real research; this has not prevented its wide-scale use in government and in health care. Perhaps more importantly, the notion of class assumes that people within a class grouping are all the same. It ignores the differences that exist between individuals and concentrates on the aspects that they have in common.

Giddens (1993:215) defines class as 'a large scale grouping of people who share common economic resources, which strongly influence the types of life style they lead'. He argues that ownership of wealth, together with occupation, is the chief basis of class difference. Theories of stratification find their origins in the work of Karl Marx and Max Weber. For Marx, class is founded on economic conditions and objectively structured economic inequalities in society. Weber argues that class divisions derive not only from control or lack of control of the means of production, but on economic and status differences, which may have nothing to do with property. Such resources include skills and credentials or qualifications that affect the type of job that people do. Weber defines two other basic aspects of stratification besides class, those of status and party. Class is relatively objective, derived from property earnings etc., but status depends on subjective evaluation of styles of life as a measure of social differences. Party defines a group of individuals who share common backgrounds, aims and interests.

A number of different ways for utilising the concept of class have been put forward, most of which are based on a person's occupation. Work continues to be closely linked to the level of income and amount of wealth as well as to skills and qualifications. Classifications based on occupations include: the social class based on occupation system (formerly known as the Registrar-General Scale), Goldthorpe's model, socio-economic groupings and, as discussed previously, various feminist models. Social classes can be defined as broad groups of people who share a similar economic situation, such as occupation, income and ownership of wealth. In Britain, the population is assigned to the various class groups by virtue of their occupation. Skills and qualifications, and an individual's standing in society, are still dictated by occupation. The unemployed therefore are seen as having no wealth, no skills, no qualifications and no status. Women who are lone mothers, supported only by state benefits, probably have the lowest status of all, apart perhaps from the disabled and those from ethnic minorities. Their contribution to society as carers and parents is frequently devalued and their very existence is the subject of regular moral panics.

There are various methods of measuring social class. Birth statistics including data on stillbirths and perinatal death are now coded using the Standard Occupational Classification. The way this is constructed is likely to change in 2002. The system in use will then become the National Statistics Socio-economic Classification. The latest figures available are still based on social class by occupation. The classification system is fraught with difficulties and in 1998 a group led by Rose and O'Reilly (1998) was commissioned to investigate the issue in depth.

In their extensive report, Rose and O'Reilly (1998) seek to address some of the problems in the classification system. The writers report on the development of a new government social classification and the development of an interim revised social classification to be used in the 2001 census. As previously discussed, the previous Registrar-General's scheme rested on the assumption that society is a graded hierarchy of occupations. This meant that occupation groups were allocated to social classes commensurate with the degree of expertise or skill in carrying out the tasks of the occupations within the groups and the resulting categories were assumed homogeneous in these terms. Midwives, along with many other health professional groups, make similar assumptions. Skill has always been seen in some part of social class. This classification has been subject to criticism (e.g. Thomas 1990) mainly because of the lack of a clear conceptual basis. Many sociologists (e.g. Edgell 1993, Nichols 1979) have questioned the idea that occupation is the key indicator of social class. Occupationally based socio-economic groups and social class divisions have become outmoded, not least because they exclude some of the most deprived groups in society. Other problems relate to the unit of analysis. Is the unit of class the individual or the family or household? If the family is the unit of analysis, the consequences of unequal distribution of resources have graver implications for women (in female hidden poverty) than men. Elias (1997:38) believes that a large number of anomalies exist with a skill-based SOC (social class based on occupation), and that revision is now essential. He contends that social statisticians will still need social class categories as a simple method for condensing the complexities of occupational structure to differentiated social groups. He warns against the simple allocation of occupations to class categories on the basis of 'some subjective notions about the skill content of occupations'. Elias favours a more rigorous and quantitative approach and argues that if the labour market rewards skills, it would seem appropriate to use information on the distribution of earnings by occupation to assist in the identification of skill levels and the allocation to SOC unit groups of broad skill categories. He believes that this would reflect significant income differences between social groupings. Although Elias' arguments were not totally accepted his points are a valid contribution to the debate on defining social class.

The interim report, produced by Rose and O'Reilly (1998), recognises that throughout industry, local and central government, the academic world and the private sector, Social Economic Classifications (SECs) are still widely used and there is a consensus of support that the ONS should continue to produce social classifications. It was argued that central and local government and government agencies still viewed social classifications as fundamental to policy formulation, targeting and evaluation. Important changes to the next census were recommended including: the need to distinguish between employees and the self-employed, and self-employed with and without employees; the need to have a question that asks about whether people manage or supervise others; and the need to have information on the numbers of employees in an establishment. The authors also argued for the need to have information on the highest qualification and to be able to distinguish those who are entirely dependent on state benefits or retirement pensions. This work led to the changes outlined in the next section. The previous relatively simple and well-known classification by occupation, which is used in the 2000 statistics, is set out below.

Social class defined by occupation

Non-manual	
I	Professional, e.g. doctors and lawyers
II	Managerial and technical occupations (teachers, most managerial and senior administrative occupations)
IIIN	Non-manual skilled occupations (clerks and shop assistants)

Manual

IIIM	Manual skilled occupations (bricklayers, underground coal miners)
IV	Partly skilled occupations (bus conductor and postman)
V	Unskilled occupations (porters and labourers)
OTHER	Residual groups such as armed forces, persons with inadequately described occupations, persons unemployed and persons with no stated occupation

The National Statistics Socio-economic Classification

In future years, statistics on birth and deaths will be presented using this new method of classification. The new classification answers many of the criticisms of the previous flawed method of assessing social class by occupation but it does mean that it will be more difficult to make comparisons from year to year. There are nine categories in the new classification.

1. Higher managerial and professional occupations
2. Lower managerial and professional occupations
3. Intermediate occupations
4. Small employers and own account workers
5. Lower supervisory and technical occupations
6. Semi-routine occupations
7. Routine occupations
8. Never worked and long-term unemployed
9. Not classified

Notions of class, whether alive or dead, remain important to the professionals who draw conclusions and in understanding the shape and the nature of society. Such issues are central in directing, shaping and developing policy. However, policy formation is formal and structuralist; it assumes that social class groups are homogeneous and that their problems can be solved by applying universal, catch-all solutions. For the women who contributed to the study, definitions, classifications and solutions were irrelevant. What was relevant was the impact of such categories and views on the quality of care they received.

DOES POVERTY MATTER? THE IMPACT OF INEQUALITIES IN HEALTH

Whatever the problems of measuring social class, it is this process which has informed the debate on the inequalities in health. In the next section, it is important to ask if poverty matters. Whilst it is clear that poverty leads to or is the end result of inequality and social deprivation, the consequences of poverty have a more profound effect on women, and in particular on childbearing women.

The link between poverty and poor health is well established both through statistics which demonstrate the inverse relationship between occupational class and mortality and morbidity and through studies which more directly link poor health, both physical and mental, to circumstances of deprivation such as damp, overcrowding, inadequate nutrition etc. (Graham 1984, Hyndman 1990, Phillimore 1989, Strachan 1986). There continue to be social divisions and inequalities of health in modern Britain; this has been borne out by the Black Report 1980 (Townsend and Davidson 1982) and subsequent other research studies (Acheson 1998, Whitehead 1988). In 1991, Clare Blackburn demonstrated the ways in which poverty affected the health of families and young children. Using qualitative and quantitative data, she demonstrated that poverty has a major impact on health and that poor health of families in poverty could not be explained simply in terms of their failure to adopt desirable attitudes to health. Despite falling stillbirth and infant mortality rates in this country, women living in poverty are still more likely to lose a baby than other women (Botting 1997). Improving the financial, social and environmental conditions of women is, according to Sir Donald Acheson (1998), likely to be an essential part of any strategy to reduce socio-economic inequalities.

The government's response to the *Independent Inquiry into Inequalities in Health Report* (Acheson 1998) was the White Paper, *Saving Lives: Our Healthier Nation* (DoH 1999), which recommended a partnership between individuals, communities and government to improve health and tackle inequalities. This was further developed in the NHS Plan with national and local targets to address inequalities. One key area for attention was a target to narrow the gap in infant and early childhood mortality and morbidity between socio-economic groups. Measuring the socio-economic status of babies is fraught with difficulties. The challenge is whether to decide the occupation or status of the mother, the father, the child or the household. Marital status is recorded but it cannot discriminate between couples who cohabit in a stable and supportive relationship and those whose partners live with them 'on and off'.

Poverty represents the extreme illustration of a socially divided society but studies of the nation's health also show the effect of social divisions. Poverty and inequality are different but are closely related. Britain, along with every other member state of the European Region of the World Health Organisation (WHO), is committed to the European Health for All Strategy, which has as its first target:

'Target 1: by the year 2000, the differences in health status between countries and between groups within countries should be reduced by twenty five per cent by improving the level of health of disadvantaged nations and groups' (WHO 1991).

Public health Green Papers have now been published in all four countries of the United Kingdom. Whilst there are differences in emphasis and approach, all recognise the fact and scale of inequalities, the link between health inequalities and wider inequalities in life chances and living standards, the need for policies which tackle broader social causes and the potential contribution of area-based interventions (Graham 1998). The Northern Ireland document (DHSS 1997) states:

'The causes of inequalities are complex and not fully understood. However, it is clear that many of the major inequalities are associated with disadvantage, whether this is measured by income, level of educational achievement or occupation. Factors which affect health and well being such as poverty, unemployment, inadequate housing, lack of social support and low educational attainment are more common in disadvantaged neighbourhoods and groups.'

The English Green Paper, *Our Healthier Nation* (DoH 1998b), recognises that people's health is affected by their circumstances. Inequalities in health have worsened in the past two decades. In this case, the literature would lead us to believe that the evidence is clear and irrefutable and it is difficult to disagree. This may well be a situation where universal solutions, in the form of a redistribution of wealth, may be entirely justified.

The latest edition of *Social Trends 32* (ONS 2002) confirms that in 1999-2000, 18 per cent of the population of Great Britain lived in households with low income (below 60 per cent of median disposable income after housing costs). This is a fall from a peak of 21 per cent in 1992. Children continue to be disproportionately represented in low-income households: in 1999-2000, 23 per cent of children, which is 3 million, were still living in households with below 60 per cent of median income in Great Britain. This is a slight improvement; in 1996-97 it was some 26 per cent.

Current benefits are still considered to be inadequate to maintain the health of childbearing women. An increase in benefits for pregnant women is essential, and age discrimination against very young pregnant women should be abolished. Single pregnant mothers in this study often went without food in the days before the benefit cheque arrived. When they did have money the local shop was generally inadequate to provide them with the components of a healthy diet at a reasonable cost. Sadly, some of the midwives who were involved in their care did not accept that the benefits were inadequate. Some midwives believed that if women were to stop smoking, drinking, adopting other deviant behaviours and spending money inappropriately, all would be well. The midwives were caught up in the belief that poverty and its consequences were solely the fault of the poor. Some believed that it was the women themselves who were solely responsible for their poverty and subsequently their ill health.

Richard Wilkinson, in his book *Unhealthy Societies* (1996), demonstrates that life expectancy in different countries is dramatically improved where income differences are smaller and societies are more socially cohesive. The greatest overall health is seen when the differential between the rich and poor is less. He suggests that if income differences were narrowed, mortality in England and Wales would improve but it would be those living in poverty that would benefit most. Wilkinson quotes Waldmann's 1992 study, which found that if the absolute incomes of the poorest 20 per cent in each society are held constant, rises in incomes of the top 5 per cent are associated with *rises* in infant mortality. It would be expected that rises in the incomes of the top 5 per cent of the richest would, all other things being held equal, have led to a reduction in infant mortality, but the opposite in fact happened. This, argues Wilkinson, is a powerful demonstration of the importance of relative income and suggests that there is a genuinely social effect of income inequality amongst poorer as well as richer countries. He also contends that the degree of inequality in modern societies 'shows the extent to which we ignore each other's welfare' (1996:143). He suggests that one of the ways that individuals in society tolerate social injustice and inequality is by assuming that an individual's position in society is a reflection of their innate worth. This is an important issue for midwives; by assuming that a woman's needs were only related to her address and social class, some midwives ignored individual needs, devalued the differences between individual women and failed to respond to the issues that arose as a result of their experience of childbirth.

Some midwives valued individuals only in relation to their position in society; some women were clearly aware of this and made strenuous efforts to appear to be respectable and thus produce a change in the midwives' attitudes.

The evidence from the literature is that poverty leads to lasting psychological and emotional damage. Poverty leads to an increase in stress and conflict, and this in turn reduces the capacity of individuals to overcome difficulties, cope with the unexpected and to maintain good health. As Wilkinson states so clearly:

'It is not just that worries about money, jobs and housing spill over into domestic conflict as tempers become more quickly frayed and parents find themselves with smaller reserves of patience and tolerance. It is also that lack of money, of choices, play space, the need for indoor space to accommodate incompatible family activities – in short, the lack of resources of all kinds (including time) – means that people's needs and demands are brought into conflict with each other. The tighter the constraints within which a family must operate, the fewer the demands which can be satisfied, and the more people's interests conflict. The smaller the resources, the less the capacity to overcome unforeseen difficulties, accidents, breakages or losses. The greater the potential sources of stress and conflict, the more family life and social support will suffer' (1996:163).

In the next section, the impact of poverty on health is further discussed. For childbearing women living in poverty the risks of their child dying or being born in poor health are significantly increased.

PERINATAL MORTALITY AND POVERTY

Perinatal and infant mortality rates show a vast variation between countries and between regions. There is clear evidence of the effects of social disadvantage in perinatal and infant mortality statistics. In 2000 the perinatal mortality rate for England and Wales was 8.0 per 1,000 live and stillbirths. However, in births where the occupation of the father is recorded, in 2000 the perinatal mortality rate varied from 6.3 in social class I to 13.7 in social class V (ONS Monitor, DH3 33 2001).

The association between lower social class and low birth weight or infant mortality is evident in the medical literature. Although many studies have simply highlighted the link or association between social factors and low birth weight, the cause is far from clear. It has been suggested that poverty could adversely affect maternal health at the time of conception (Howe *et al.* 1985, Leiberman 1995) and that less healthy women are more likely to be found in lower social classes. The medical literature, unsurprisingly, tends to support explanations such as variation in the quality of medical care, diet, poor housing, lower social support, increased exposure to toxic agents or increased risk of infectious diseases (Mutale *et al.* 1991).

Rutter and Quine (1990) consider four theories to explain the link between social factors and adverse pregnancy outcomes. The first, known as the artefact theory, suggests that the association is merely as a result of the ways in which social class is defined. Longitudinal studies, for example the National Child Development Survey, would seem to refute this theory. The second, 'natural or social selection', suggests that unhealthy people select or drift towards low-status occupations, whilst healthy people drift upwards. This argument was rejected in the Black Report, the findings of which were well hidden by the government of the day. The third theory states that material deprivation affects health directly. The fourth theory says that material deprivation works indirectly either through individual behaviour, lack of medical services or a poor diet. Rutter and Quine suggest that the third and fourth theories should be examined together as material deprivation, culture and behaviour. Somewhat arrogantly they suggest that people at the bottom of the social scale suffer material deprivation and are part of a culture in which predominant forms of health behaviour, such as smoking, are considered harmful. The culture of poverty argument is also made suggesting that material deprivation itself produces 'inappropriate behaviour'.

Dunn (1984) suggests that the influence of social class may be exerted through intermediate factors which may be biological (such as maternal weight, parity and age) or environmental (like smoking, stress and poor take-up of medical care). The relationship between social class and low birth weight has been demonstrated consistently to exist across time, geographical areas and definitions of social class. What is unknown is exactly how social factors translate into the physical and biological mechanisms that adversely affect pregnancy.

The mechanisms that clarify the connections between poor health and social class are not yet clearly identified. The fact that such links exist is important and relevant to this research. The evidence that has been presented thus far serves to illustrate the nature and sources of knowledge that is available to midwives. It is not surprising therefore that midwives see themselves as superior, more knowledgeable and disgruntled in having to deal with women they consider deviant and non-compliant.

DIET, PREGNANCY AND POVERTY

In the government's report on *Inequalities in Health*, Acheson (1998) states that mothers reliant on state benefits may not be able to afford a healthy diet and may go short in order to feed their children (see also Dobson *et al.* 1994, Dowler and Calvert 1995). Yet, in the United States, guaranteeing a minimum income to pregnant women has been shown to increase birth weight. This is a universal solution that may have some benefit – not least that an increase in state benefits would provide some choice for women who are struggling with poverty.

The Maternity Alliance's research, *Poor Expectations* (1995), has also shown that many pregnant women on supplementary benefit are incapable of affording a healthy diet. The greater likelihood of women from ethnic minorities to live in deprived areas and be in poverty renders them more likely to suffer from an inadequate diet and low health standard. Equally, mothers in low-income groups are more likely to smoke and less likely to breast-feed. The 1990 OPCS survey on breast-feeding showed that this continues to be a social class-related activity. In Britain, older and more educated women were most likely to breast-feed: 78 per cent of babies from professional classes compared with only 51 per cent from manual workers' families. Many studies have demonstrated the link between social deprivation, smoking and low birth weight (Milham and Davis 1991, Sexton and Hebel 1984). More recently it has been suggested that fetal under-nutrition can lead to increased cardiovascular disease and diabetes in middle age (Fall *et al.* 1995, Hales *et al.* 1991). Premature birth and poor fetal growth are a major cause of death during the perinatal and neonatal periods.

For women, obesity is more common in lower social classes: 25 per cent of women in social class V are obese compared with 14 per cent in social class I (Prescott-Clarke and Primatesta 1998). The children of women who are overweight are at increased risk of coronary heart disease as adults (Forsen *et al.* 1997). For the women in this study, a healthy diet was often unobtainable. As Dobson *et al.* (1994) have demonstrated, the food budget was one area of expenditure that was reduced in order to meet unexpected and immediate demands. Similarly, healthy-eating messages are often lost, although families received information about food and food-related issues from a variety of sources. The implementation of food-related health messages was often not considered feasible simply because of limited resources. Dobson *et al.* (1994) found that the 'discipline of poverty fell most heavily on mothers to the extent that they often ceased to derive pleasure from eating'. They worked to protect their children from the effects of a low income, often sacrificing their own food preferences in the process. The realities of life on a low income mean that women cannot buy in bulk or plan food purchases in advance. Buying even cheaper food was often the only way of managing an unexpected bill. The sign in the local supermarket alongside the frozen chips section was an accurate reflection of the diet. It said: 'Due to the high demand for this product, purchases are limited to six bags per customer.' The staple diet of many families was inexpensive, high-fat food.

In Hilary Graham's study of lone mothers (1987a) she describes how women living with men adapt their own food preferences to those of their partners. Although women take the major responsibility for the preparation of the family's meals, they do not determine the content. In one-parent families, children's food preferences remained important. Once separated from their partners, women had greater control over what to buy and what to cook, but it also presented them with the opportunity to economise more on food. For some of the women in this study, going without was the way in which they managed an income that was insufficient. The other major strategy was to avoid waste by eating whatever the children had left. Obesity was the inevitable consequence of an inadequate diet, a lack of expensive fresh foods and eating habits that involved 'grazing' on leftovers.

I felt that coping with domestic violence, managing the money, feeding the family and crime were the main sources of stress to some of the women in the study. From this section, it is clear poverty does matter. The evidence is convincing that poverty has an adverse effect on the health of individuals and the population. However, what is also important is the impact of poverty amongst childbearing women on some midwives' attitudes to, and perception of, the needs of women living in poverty.

PREGNANCY, POVERTY AND THE HEALTH PROFESSIONAL: SOME WOMEN'S EXPERIENCES OF MATERNITY CARE

All of the women in this study were pregnant and had a baby during the fieldwork stage of the study. Over half, 16 out of 25, had experienced ill health in the previous year. From backache to depression, from epilepsy to cancer of the cervix, the women were familiar with ill health and familiar with the process of seeking help and advice from health professionals. They distrusted the health service. Most had changed their GP in the previous year, but had adopted an attitude of acceptance of what they believed was an inferior service. They felt that many hospital midwives did not approve of them, their life styles or the choices that they made about their lives. They seemed to distrust authority and resented the 'interfering busy bodies' who tried to exert control over their lives. Health visitors, midwives and doctors' receptionists were openly criticised and verbally abused. People who were thought to be in authority were resented and generally seen as the enemy. It took a considerable amount of time to reassure the women that I was not from the council, the 'social', the social services or some other source of power or control. The women I interviewed were acutely aware of the power that others could have over their lives. In this example, Carol shares her views and explains how she feels health professionals use and abuse their powers.

Carol [20] said:

'I have changed my GP three times; they won't come out at night. They think that the likes of us aren't worth it. Whatever the problem is the receptionist says bring 'em down to the surgery. That's okay if you've got a car, but how do you bring one sick kid down, wrapped in a blanket, with three others in tow. If they are sick, I'll soon be bringing them out at night. It's the same with them all. You come to the surgery. I bet they don't say that to posh folks with cars. And when you go they blame me if he's ill. It's because I smoke or it's because I don't give them the right food. It's always my fault, never theirs. If the doctor does not know what's wrong, it's never his fault. They think they are perfect.

The health visitors are the worst, always sticking their noses in, telling me how to look after my children. One at the surgery does not even have any kids herself. A right know it all.'

In the next extract, I explore some of the practical effects of poverty, and the interaction between these women in poverty and the medical profession. I found this to be a deeply disturbing episode and one where I could not confine myself to the role of researcher. I spoke with Kirsty's [21] grandmother. Kirsty's son had been born with talipes equinovarus, or clubfoot. This is when both feet are bent downwards and inwards. At the time of the interview the boy was five years old and had started school. It was impossible to find him shoes that fitted: one foot was two sizes bigger than the other and buying two pairs of shoes was out of the question. He had gym shoes but did not go to school on rainy days. I asked what the consultant orthopaedic surgeon had advised and how his treatment was progressing. His grandmother explained that he had been seen at the local hospital as a baby, but no treatment had been planned. She told me that she was always anxious about doctors. 'I suppose they know what they're doing, but I don't trust them really,' she said. I asked when he was next due to see an orthopaedic consultant, but his grandmother said that they had been told by the GP to wait until he was sent for. This family – Kirsty, a single mother with three children, and her mother – simply accepted this explanation. There was no health visitor contact and like many families Kirsty and her family had changed addresses on many occasions. I found it impossible not to become involved; I explained that they should seek an urgent orthopaedic appointment through their GP. I wrote the details on a sheet of paper and spoke with the GP. Within a week, Kirsty's son was seen in a children's hospital and had corrective surgery three weeks later. Some six months later, her son was walking with much greater ease and his mother was able to buy him shoes. A lack of knowledge, and acceptance of the system, had led to this boy being at a disadvantage. If the family had confidence in their GP and felt it was their right as customers to complain and question it is unlikely that they would have accepted this situation for such a protracted period. Anger and resentment against the power and authority of the professionals was not easily translated into action. In this situation the woman and her mother had neither the knowledge nor the power to resolve the dilemma.

The women in this study did what they could: changed GPs frequently, moved house frequently, failed to attend appointments, refused to answer the door to the health visitor and called at the surgery when they knew the receptionist had gone home. But communication is a two-way process; these women knew when the professionals engaged with them and when they kept the emotional, spiritual and physical door closed. They were not able to orchestrate a change in either the attitudes or the actions of the health professionals who so often failed to walk alongside them. The opportunity to capitalise on the energy and willingness of these women was lost. A new partnership which embraces, befriends and walks alongside, sharing human contact with knowledge, experience and professional judgement, is essential if anything is to improve.

Kirsty [21] said:

'I am pretty fed up with them at the hospital. They are all the same they treat women like me as if they were a nuisance. Always bothering them and always causing trouble. Then if I don't turn up at the clinic that's wrong too. There is always something I've done wrong. It's not true. Some midwives are okay but the others treat me and people like me as if I am a nuisance to them.

Sometimes I struggle to get to the hospital and then they just keep you waiting. I am sure other women get called in before me. They just look at you, turn their noses up and keep you waiting. They think you have a car waiting outside. That's a joke.'

Judy [17] said:

'I always make an effort to look tidy when I go to the

hospital. They like you better if you are clean and tidy, you know looking respectable like. The midwife at home says it doesn't matter, but it does. Once I thought I would use a different address to see if they treated me any better but I couldn't get my head around it.'

Tammy [13] was a 17-year-old single woman, experiencing her first pregnancy. She was a very small, pale-looking woman with very long hair that hung over much of her face. She was shy and at first reluctant to talk to me. She often looked away during the conversations but gradually she began to trust me more, and later, during subsequent meetings, she spoke at length about her experiences following the premature birth of her son. This is what she said:

'The community midwives are great but I don't like the hospital ones. At least they listen to me. I always felt they had some respect for me. The hospital ones are the problem. Too busy, or pretending to be too busy. Never stopping to listen or find out about you. Because I was young (I was only seventeen when he was born) and single they thought I couldn't look after him. He was in special care for four weeks. The nurses there were horrible, my Mum put a letter of complaint in, it were only little things, you know. They sell baby creams, they would ask all the other Mums but not ask me. It was the little things.

I was different. They wouldn't let me do anything with him; they wouldn't let me change him or anything. They would do it, but I found out all the other mothers were doing their own. They just didn't trust me to look after him, but I was the one going to take him home. They looked down their noses at me, as if I was something they trod on. Always criticising. It was always as if they didn't approve.

They would say things like "do you think you can get here to feed him by 10 o'clock". Well of course I could, it was as if they thought I couldn't look after him, it was great when I came home.

The community midwives were great. They kept saying I was doing a good job. A would smile at me and say I was a lovely little mother. That was really nice. My Mum said that too. And he's all right.'

Although midwifery prides itself on the delivery of individualised care, for both Tammy and Kirsty, these hospital midwives made judgements about her care based on their own perception of her needs. These midwives appeared to fail to recognise the issues inherent in the power of the professional operating in her own territory, i.e. the hospital. *Changing Childbirth* (DoH 1993), still the policy document guiding care in the maternity services, advocates choice, control, continuity of care and effective communication. Kirsty had little choice, no control over the events, no continuity of care or carer until she came home, and ineffective communication because nobody listened to what she wanted or tried to find out what she already knew or could do.

In another example, Lisa [14], a 20-year-old woman having her second baby, described her childbirth experiences:

'The community midwives are okay, no trouble with them at all, but the hospital midwives are no good. You just feel stupid the way they talk to you. I went in with bad pains and they said "oh its nothing" and sent me home. Some of the young ones who ain't had kids themselves and think they know it all, I don't like that. I was in agony. This young midwife comes in and says "you're all right". I thought how does she know. The woman next door was in serious pain. They gave her nothing. She has not had a child herself; they don't know what they are talking about. I trust the old uns, even if they have not had a baby, but I don't trust the young uns. I don't like them, they haven't got the experience. It's just the way they speak to you really. It's as if they don't approve of you. I felt that all the time. They were always just palming me off. They were just not kind.'

There is an ongoing debate in midwifery as to the relevance of a personal experience of childbirth in providing good midwifery care. Just as it is not necessary to have a heart attack to care for someone with this condition, good midwifery care does not depend on the midwife having had a child. Indeed such an experience may be detrimental to care if, for example, her own experience had been that of an easy birth. However, it is a reasonable point of reference for women trying to make sense of the maternity services and illustrates the women's frustration with a system of care that does not respond to their needs.

Claire [24], a 38-year-old divorcee with three children, had similar complaints. Whilst she described the care offered by the community midwives as 'great' she was clearly dissatisfied with hospital-based care. She said:

'The community midwives are great. But when you go into labour, when you have got three kids already they say "let her get on with it". You know leave her. They look at your address, see [name of street] and treat you as if you are nothing. It does not matter how many kids you have had, you are still scared when you go into labour. They didn't bother with me for hours. They left me in a room on my own for hours. My partner came for a bit, but he had to go and look after the others. I said to them, "look my waters have gone". The midwife said "well yes, just leave it, it's all right, you know what you are doing, I'll let you get on with it". I felt like getting up and smacking her one. They treat you as if you were something like dirt.

I don't like these trainee ones around me either, you are in labour, they are poking around asking daft questions and then they don't listen to the answers. It's daft when you are in pain. When you have a lot of kids they just leave you alone. They think you are used to it. They shouldn't do that. I wanted a home birth, with the community midwife, but the hospital said, because I had had a slight stroke I should come in, but was the point when they left me alone all the time?'

The perception of being 'treated like dirt' or 'something that they trod on' was a common one. Some women defined themselves as poor: 'Of course I am not rich, there just isn't enough money to go around, so I must be poor,' one said. It was clear, however, that being poor and pregnant was not a problem but the attitude of midwives was a problem. Some women felt that their social standing adversely influenced their care, by their address and by their obvious material disadvantage. They felt that their care was not as good as it should have been and they felt that they were powerless to do anything about it.

As previously discussed there is an issue in the social sciences about the relationship between *structures* as definitions of reality and *agency*, the experience of individuals, and which is more significant. Most commentators, e.g. Giddens (1984), believe that such definitions are outdated and there is a place and a clear need for a combination of both. The social, economic and political contexts have shaped the lives of women like Claire, but her individual agency, her experience and how she responds to experiences have also shaped her views. The views and actions of some midwives were similarly shaped, by both the structures of society and their own experiences. Claire, like other women in the study, did not feel that she warranted special attention because she was materially poor, but she did object to being the victim of stereotyping and labelling. She knew that the midwives were marginalising her and that she was dismissed when she complained. However, the type of care she wanted was exactly the same as a woman from any other social group. She wanted good care, support from a non-judgemental, competent midwife and effective communication. She wanted to feel as if she was in control of what was happening to her and she wanted the ability to have a say in her care. The community midwives acknowledged her as a person, gave her the information she needed to make choices and supported her through the childbirth process. The hospital midwives she met, far from supporting her, chose to demonstrate that they had greater power than she had in that setting. It appears that some community midwives at least were capable of seeing women beyond their class labels and beyond their status and position as determined by their address and postal code. Some midwives were able to see women as individuals, different women with different needs. Sadly, others could not and were determined to make judgements about women and 'fix' people in terms of their social class and place. The issues of territory (hospital versus home) and the power that goes with the owner of the space are important but more important is the willingness of the professional to engage, to provide human contact, even if just for a moment, with the woman wherever she might be. A human dimension to the encounter and a real willingness to engage with the woman as a human being is crucial.

Barbara [10] was a 36-year-old mother of three, whose complaints about the maternity services were even more specific. Her fourth child was delivered by caesarean section following a difficult birth. She argued that the midwife was not assertive enough and did not convince her of the importance of changing her position in labour. She said:

'When I was in labour, I had Pethidine. It makes you high, the midwife suggested I went on my hands and knees to help the baby turn. Someone who is high on Pethidine needs more direction. It's as if they have gone soft. I wanted her to do more than suggest. I needed to know how important it was. I needed a reason not a suggestion.

When you are in pain you need direction. It could have made a difference the baby could have turned.

It's not about being in control; the midwife is in control, she knows more than me. It's about saying what's important. She didn't manage to do that. It doesn't matter who you are, if you are rich or poor, when you are in labour and things are going wrong you need the best person there is to take care of you and show the way. That's what any woman deserves.'

Barbara, along with other women, praised the work of the community midwives. She explained that these midwives were not 'bossy' like the hospital midwives and seemed to have more time to talk and explain things to the women. Community midwives, perhaps because they were used to the women and the area, were not seen as judgemental, neither did they make pejorative remarks like their hospital-based colleagues. Community midwives work in GPs' surgeries, health centres and women's own homes. The territory belongs to the woman; it is her space and to some extent the midwife is a guest. The location of care may influence the balance of power in the relationship. The majority of the women saw them as kind, supportive friends who were acceptable and who could make time for them. Hospital midwives work under difficult conditions: they are more likely to be short-staffed and working under pressure; they do not have the same opportunity to establish relationships with women as do the community midwives.

Emma [25], a 15-year-old single woman, summed up her feelings about the community midwives like this:

'I like A ... you can ask her anything at all. She explains it all, tells you what's happening and doesn't make you feel stupid. I was really scared of labour till I talked to A. She treated me well, she said you can have this, ask for that, you know. You don't have to stay in bed if you don't want to, you can walk around, go in the bath that really helped. When I went in I felt, as I was in charge not them, A helped a lot.

She said you can say if you only want a low dose of Pethidine to start. They come and see you at home, you just have to leave a message at the surgery, they don't

have a go at you for smoking. They are just kind really. The hospital ones have a go all the time.

It appears that community midwives were better able to establish a relationship with childbearing women than their hospital-based colleagues. All midwives had the opportunity to exert power over women and in so doing make or mar their childbearing experience. They also had the opportunity to share that power with women by giving them information and discussing options with them. Some chose not to share any of their power.

DIFFERENT WOMEN, DIFFERENT EXPERIENCES, DIFFERENT PROBLEMS: POVERTY, LIFE STYLE AND THE MIDWIFE'S VIEWS

In my conversations with both hospital and community midwives, it became clear that many hospital midwives thought that poor women should not have children. Although they were sometimes embarrassed by their own views, once I had established a relationship with them, the midwives I met were willing to express these views, albeit anonymously. At a hospital staff meeting, called to discuss the health authority's health action zone bid, I was party to a number of informal conversations. I was also able to make detailed notes of public comments and views expressed by both hospital and community-based midwives. It became clear that some midwives believed that the women I was working with were feckless, inadequate and even stupid, as well as a drain on the country's resources. It was also clear that midwives had little idea about how women living in poverty made choices. When a woman living in poverty spent money on cigarettes, drugs or alcohol they were ridiculed and their choices condemned. These are some of the comments that some midwives made, which were either recorded or noted soon after the meeting:

'How can they be poor when they always have money to spend on cigarettes, "a four pack" [of beer], and they all have televisions and videos. I don't know why they have children, they can't look after them, feed them, or buy them the things they need.'

'If you give them more money they will only spend it on beer and cigarettes. They can't look after their children as it is. It's my tax that goes to pay for them to lie about, smoke, drink and get pregnant.'

'We spend hours telling them how to eat properly. What food to buy, what is good for them and the baby. What do they do? Live on chips and fags. It's a waste of my time and effort. They never breast-feed, don't take iron and never take advice.'

'They are all the same. Scroungers, a drain on the system. They do not come to clinic. They always default and then we spend time running around after them. Their babies are small. They spend weeks in special care, more time, more resources. I know one consultant who says they should put the pill in the drinking water in that area, that would save us all a lot of trouble.'

These midwives demonstrated their intolerance and poor understanding of the complexities of living in material deprivation. They failed to see women as individuals with individual needs. They made assumptions about their life styles and about their spending decisions. They failed to see beyond their own prejudices and stereotypes.

Hilary Graham (1987b, 1993) has worked extensively with women living in material deprivation; she found clear links between smoking (amongst white women), their having caring responsibilities and living in material deprivation. She says:

'The limited evidence suggests that cigarette smoking is deeply woven into the strategies women develop to cope with caring and to survive in circumstances of hardship. In talking about smoking in the context of poverty, material hardship gives them and their children little opportunity to take part in life styles that others take for granted. They are unlikely to be able to afford either major new clothes or travelling out with their partner. In a life style with little style left in it, smoking cigarettes can be the only item of personal spending and the only luxury' (Graham 1993).

Of women who contributed to this study, 15 out of 25 were smokers. Some had tried to give up during their pregnancy; others only smoked outside or when the children had gone to bed; but the remainder confirmed Hilary Graham's explanation. Smoking was one of the few things that women could do for themselves; it represented relaxation, pleasure in a harsh existence, peace and quiet, a release of stress. The health risks were distant and remote and the satisfaction immediate. Emma [25] explained:

'Fags are good to relax. After a hard day with the kids, I like to curl up with a fag. I only smoke when the kids are outside or after they have gone to bed. I know it's not good for them, but it's good for me, it helps me unwind.'

I was not surprised by the views held by these midwives, having heard such opinions articulated at conferences and seminars for some years. But why do midwives behave as they do? Where are their assumptions based? What analysis have they made and what conclusions do they draw? Some midwives appear to believe that some women are poor because they smoke; they are seen as irresponsible, they waste their money, do not eat properly, do not follow their advice and generally behave inadequately. They fail to use contraception, neglect the children they have and through their own inadequacies get themselves into difficulties. Some midwives appear to believe that women living in poverty have a choice and could choose a better life style if they wished. However, this is an oversimplification. It assumes that poor women are all the same and that they are all uniformly responsible for their situation. It ignores the differences between individual women and ignores the diverse factors that have contributed to their poverty. It is clear that some midwives believe they are superior to these women. They practise midwifery according to their model and philosophy of poverty. Some midwives appear to believe that all women living in poverty are sick and are at risk of having a child born small, ill or unwell or who will die an untimely cot death because they smoke. These beliefs lead some midwives to the erroneous conclusion that *all* poor women are inadequate and worthy of blame. The care they give then reflects these assumptions. Some midwives also believe that women smoke because they are poor and are poor because they smoke.

The positivist research reported in this chapter confirms the view that some poor women do indeed adopt inappropriate behaviour, but it ignores the fact that many do not. It is important to ponder on the fact that all social classes, all groups, have individuals who adopt inappropriate behaviour. Some rich women doubtlessly overeat, smoke cannabis, snort cocaine, drink too much and take insufficient exercise! And some of course do not. Some midwives also believe that some women living in poverty do not eat properly. This may be because their income is insufficient or because they are incapable of making 'correct choices'. Some women do eat 'properly'; they go to considerable lengths to find inexpensive and nutritious food. This is far more difficult to achieve on an inadequate income. Some midwives also believe that because some women smoke they do not worry about their health and do not care for their children in an appropriate way. When they become ill or their children are ill they are seen to be demanding even more care, which midwives consider unfair. The midwives act out their discontent on the women themselves. The women try to compensate for this discontent by adopting what they see as appropriate behaviour. Some make an effort to be 'clean and tidy' and take other steps to be seen as 'respectable', but they are faced with what is often an impossible task.

This dichotomy is based on fundamental assumptions about class and poverty. The structuralist argument states that the poor will always be with us. This leads some midwives to treat women living in poverty as the lowest of the low. The reality is that many women cannot escape from poverty yet they face the resentment of midwives who have concluded that the poor have a choice. Midwives find themselves in a dilemma: publicly and subjectively they believe in choice but objectively believe in 'truth'. The truth they see is that women are poor by choice, the poverty leads to ill health and they conclude that ill health is the fault of the poor and construct their care accordingly.

This research has clearly demonstrated the flaw in this argument. Throughout the study, I have been able to show that there is no such thing as uniform behaviour, no life style that reflects social class groupings. Indeed, I have demonstrated that there is no universal experience of poverty, no universal response to violence, no universal reason for smoking and for not smoking. In this study, I found that women were very different. What they shared in common was poverty, but the ways in which they experienced poverty and coped with the effects of poverty varied from woman to woman. It is clear that many people smoke, from all social classes, but it is women living in poverty who fall under the judgement of the midwives. Some midwives who see themselves as belonging to a superior, more educated class look down on women living in poverty who smoke and openly criticise their actions.

The search for professional status, even the move into higher education, may have led some midwives to distance themselves from some pregnant women, in particular the types of women who have contributed to this study. Negotiation and partnership needs a belief in equality and equity. For some women such a partnership and belief system did not exist. Midwives can gain knowledge and experience from the women in their care. Although pregnancy and labour often follow a similar pattern, it is still an individual process experienced by individual women. Only if the feelings of individuals are listened to, and then shared with colleagues, will the body of midwives' knowledge be increased, and the 'seeing [of] women through the eyes of experts or through stereotypes' (Kroll 1996:185) be reduced. Different cultural backgrounds are often treated with suspicion or even dislike and such stereotypes persist in midwifery settings (see for example the work of Bowler 1993). Hospital and community midwives are not inherently narrow-minded, but they are part of a society in which stereotypes and negative assumptions about people from minority cultures abound. Midwives perpetuate structures and stereotypes as a means of control and superiority. There is a clear need to acknowledge that they as midwives are individuals and can act differently from other midwives and that the women they care for are also individuals. There is also a need to acknowledge that they have the power to change the experience of childbearing women.

It is also important to consider here that the women who contributed to the study were similarly judgemental and assumed that all (hospital-based) midwives were the same. The power to alter this assumption rests with the midwives alone. As Foucault (1983:221) has said, 'power is exercised by free subjects only over free subjects and only in so far as they are free'. Power is everywhere; it is exercised not given, and at some level available to all. The midwife as the professional can use her knowledge/power to correct the inequality in care that the women describe.

I believe that midwives should try to distance themselves from the assumptions that all women are the same. They should stand back from the medical research that seeks to blame the adverse effects of poverty on the women themselves and should acknowledge openly that women are different. Recognising diversity, acknowledging difference and giving women care according to their individual needs has been a message in midwifery for many years. What this study has demonstrated is that childbearing women living in poverty are indeed very different and need individual care from the health professionals and that the messages of the midwifery literature have been ignored by some midwives.

SUMMARY

In this chapter, I have explored the concept of social class and have considered the reasons why some midwives and others appear to place such emphasis on what they believe to be the social class position and thus life style of individual women. Although class is sometimes not considered a valid analytical category and is even considered irrelevant in much postmodern theorising, it is still valuable in considering the effects of inequalities in health. Understanding class is therefore important in understanding health and in understanding how the attitudes of midwives and others are shaped by their own understanding of class.

In this chapter, I have thus considered the use of social class in defining and measuring inequalities in health and how the concept of social class can be misused by midwives and others to the detriment of some women. I have briefly explored some of the literature that demonstrates the marked social divisions that exist in the UK and the established links between poverty and ill health. I have concluded that poverty does indeed matter. Not only does poverty have adverse effects on both mental and physical health, it frequently dictates the quality of care that some midwives provide for some women. I have considered certain aspects of the relationships between some midwives and some women and I have explored the use and abuse of power and knowledge when care was based on assumptions of social class and assumed worth. I have explained why some midwives perpetuate structures and stereotypes as a means of exerting power and control over women. I have discussed how theories of social class rely on social groupings, which assume that everyone within that group is the same.

In the final chapter, I will draw together the findings of this study and consider some recommendations for changing the practice of midwifery for the better.

9

Where next?

What do we know?   Conclusions and recommendations
Recommendations for practice   for further research

WHAT DO WE KNOW?

The purpose of this ethnographic study was to understand the nature of the experiences of a small group of childbearing women living in material poverty. The study was set in the West Midlands in an area of urban decay and social deprivation. In this study, I was interested in how women as individuals made sense of their lives and their experiences of pregnancy, childbirth and motherhood; I was also interested in how women were alike and how they were different. I had interest in the similarities and what was significant about both the similarities and differences. The more I have learned the more I realise how little I know about childbearing women who live in poverty. I have looked at one pebble on the beach, I have studied that pebble in great depth, but there are layers untouched and many other pebbles. This study has provided a greater insight into the lives of childbearing women living in poverty. It has uncovered issues in the lives of individuals that only an ethnographic empirical study can. It has demonstrated that there is more than just one way of seeing, and my way, the way of midwives and perhaps the way of these women themselves are neither right nor better than any other.

The women who contributed to this study were part of a society where structures have had an impact on their lives. From Beveridge to the Third Way to *Changing Childbirth* (DoH 1993), all childbearing women have been subjected to changing government policy and a range of state interventions aimed at improving their lives. Yet, within these structural influences, there are individuals. There is a Tracey, Rachel, Mel and a Barbara. The effectiveness of any structure or structural change depends on the interaction and understanding of the individual. This study has looked beyond the structures, beyond the rules and systems, and focused on increasing an awareness of individuals and the impact of those structures on individuals. The structures form the framework of the lives of these childbearing women living in poverty. GPs and midwives act as gateways to the structures but each woman has used her own agency to find ways of surviving within the structures. The women have found ways to manage their money, manage the housing and benefit office, manage their GP, sometimes even coerce the midwives into giving better care, and to survive. Whilst the government, through targets and quotas, seeks to improve the nation's health and health care, individual women use these structures to complement, rather than dictate, their survival.

In this study I have concentrated on the individual; I have used a feminist poststructuralist framework to look beyond the structures to the lives of individuals. In adopting a poststructural analysis, there is always the danger of losing touch with the impact of structures on individuals or forgetting the big picture. By focusing too deeply on the detail of individuals and their lives, there is always the risk of ignoring the context of their lives. There is also a danger of believing that because there are no universal problems and no universal solutions that state intervention of any type is invalid and that change of whatever type rarely results in improvements for individuals. Poverty researchers are frequently structuralists and seek evidence to persuade governments to seek universal solutions. Poststructural analysis can deter response and even discourage governments from intervening. There is also the inevitable difficulty that I experienced of having to consolidate my feminist desire to find an emancipatory solution and my intellectual desire to construct a pure poststructuralist analysis. As Francis (1999:391) states:

'While we may agree theoretically that the self is constituted through discourse, we still feel ourselves to have agency, moral obligations, and preferences for different kinds of discourse; and creating narratives to structure, or describe our lives, is part of being a human subject.'

As a feminist, I wanted to find universal solutions, solve the problems and put things right yet I was able to recognise that it was the individual nature of these women that prevented me from doing so.

Hart *et al.* (2001) consider the important debate between structures and individuals. They acknowledge that social, economic and political contexts play a major role in structuring individuals' lives. They also recognise that individuals play a role in defining and shaping both their own experiences and ultimately the structures that seek to define them. They use the example of women with physical disabilities and argue that midwives, in order to offer appropriate care, must remain aware of both structural and individual aspects of disadvantage. They say:

'They [midwives] may draw on macro studies employing epidemiological and statistical data to enhance awareness of possible structural inequalities (economic, social, and/or cultural) faced by, for example, physically disabled women. However, they may need to draw on microsociological research to enable them to remain open to the possibility that individual disabled women may experience their disabilities in vastly different ways. Only by drawing on both approaches can midwives deliver appropriate care' (Hart *et al.* 2001:32)

The research presented in this book is a 'microsociological' study that demonstrates that women living in poverty experience their poverty 'in vastly different ways'. Midwives need the major studies and the data on inequalities in health but they also need to draw on studies such as this to offer the best care.

In essence, this book is about counteracting and balancing the overemphasis on structures and providing a greater understanding of the impact of poverty on individuals and on their lives. It recognises and values individual agency within existing structures. Throughout the research, I have found that there was no single unified women's voice; there was no clearly defined experience of childbirth and poverty. However, there were common themes and some shared experiences. There were similarities in experiences but differences in the ways in which women responded to these experiences. The women who contributed to this study shared a strong sense of responsibility towards their children. There was clear evidence of these women and their mothers, the grandmothers, putting children first. There was also a strong need to do what was 'right' and to be seen as respectable. I failed to find a 'truth' about women living in poverty; I cannot describe a universal experience and neither can I offer a universal solution. I have found evidence of power and knowledge being used in tandem; I have seen women exercising their power in situations where they may be described as powerless. I have seen many different shades of what I regard to be oppression and I have seen individual women respond to this oppression as both victims and survivors.

I have considered the findings of this ethnography in both the national and local framework, I have given attention to the complexities of defining and measuring poverty and I have drawn on the overwhelming evidence that demonstrates that the effects of poverty on health are significant. At the time of the study the health gap between the rich and the poor and between the north and the south of Britain was wider than ever before. In 1999, Daniel Dorling, author of a new report, 'The Widening Gap', stated that health inequalities have widened since the 1950s with infant mortality rates at least twice as high in poor areas of Britain as compared with the more prosperous areas. Death rates of children are as much as two and a half times higher in poor areas. In the worst health areas, there are 4.2 times as many children living in poverty.

Howarth *et al.* (1998) have devised a complex and multifaceted tool to monitor the effects of poverty. This tool, which can be regularly updated, is being used to monitor trends and assess progress towards the targets set by the government. They will produce a regular Poverty and Social Exclusion Report to inform the public and increase awareness and understanding of the extent and nature of the problems suffered by a significant minority of the population. The key measures, 46 in all, cover matters related to poverty and social exclusion. The measures are more concerned with the effects of poverty rather than simply measuring levels of income and expenditure. Howarth *et al.* state:

'No single indicator could possibly capture the complexity of poverty and social exclusion. Indeed as a measure of well-being, income is inadequate on its own. It takes no account of health or freedom or achievement. It does not measure happiness' (1998:17).

Rahman *et al.* (2001), using the new and revised indicators, discuss the latest statistics available. This report now shows that, for the first time, the number of indicators that improved over the latest year clearly exceeds the number that have deteriorated. One of the key indicators is the number of people living in households with less than 60 per cent of median income. The number of people living in households below 60 per cent of median income had reduced from 13.4 million in 1998-99 to 13.3 million in 1990-2000. Children continue to be more likely than adults to live in low-income households. Although there are improvements in educational standards substantial numbers still fail to obtain any qualifications at all. Housing is continuing to improve but the number of people living in temporary accommodation is still rising sharply. Accidental deaths of children, suicides amongst young adults and underage pregnancies are falling but there are still marked and persistent inequalities in health between social classes. Women in social classes IIM and V are still more likely to have low birth-weight babies than those in social classes I to IIINM. (The difficulties of recording births and deaths according to the father's occupation are discussed in earlier chapters.) Babies of lone parents are more likely to be of low birth weight than babies of couples (Rahman *et al.* 2001).

Statistics can be debated, discussed and analysed at length. Some things are getting better; some indicators show a standstill or deterioration. The structural solutions are having some effect and there are many more improvements still in the pipeline. But in this study I am drawn back to the individual; through this research, I have demonstrated something of the complexity of poverty. I have shown how poverty is experienced in different ways by different individuals and how poverty affects women as mothers and as recipients of health care.

The Chancellor, along with the Prime Minister, still searches for universal solutions. This is the nature of government. The government continues to assert that work rather than increased benefits and the redistribution of wealth are the solutions to the nation's poverty. There is little evidence that women's poverty is a separate and different issue. Structures are important: without government intervention there would be no redistribution of wealth, or universal state benefits, which help many women but still manage to miss the needs of others. As the structure of the household has changed and the proportion of families headed by a lone parent has increased, many women have become more independent but poorer. As this study has demonstrated, there are new patterns of poverty and inequality for women outside the labour market. Although much of the data for this study was collected before the 2001 general election, the prospects for the children of women living in poverty are still very difficult.

In this research, I have demonstrated how individual women and their children experience the most adverse effects of poverty at first hand.

John Grieve Smith, an economist at Robinson College, Cambridge, believes that targeting those in most need is still the most economical way of helping the poor; it also keeps down government expenditure and taxation (1999:5). Publicly, the government is opposed to the redistribution of wealth (its major increases in child benefit payments were kept fairly low key) and its mantra of 'work for those who can' and 'benefits for those who cannot' continues to be the thrust of its social policy. But work is not the answer for all women, neither is it the answer for most of the women in this study; they cannot work when they are in the latter stages of pregnancy or when they are working caring for small children. The cost of child care far exceeds anything they could earn in the local factories or shops. To reiterate the policy of work is inhumane and ignores the very real needs of childbearing women. A structural approach to poverty ignores individual needs; it ignores Tracey struggling with Christmas and the demands of a consumerism and designer labels. In this study it was possible to see how complex are individual lives and how individuals can be neglected in great reforms. Structures, great social reforms, redistribution of wealth, and new 'community schemes' are valuable but they do not always get it right and can frequently miss the individual woman on a Middleton or other housing estate. The temptation to 'play God' and convince 'the beach' that you are helping the 'whole beach' means that individual pebbles are left with no solution. This study is unique because it demonstrates that within structural solutions there continue to be individuals for whom the solution is yet to arrive.

Poverty as a concept remains contentious. Its definition continues to be subject to intense debate and controversy. Some writers, e.g. Roll (1992), believe that it is patronising to define other people as poor, whilst others feel that the stigma of poverty in this society is so great that many would deny its existence. When I was working with women I used the term *'finding it hard to make ends meet'*. I avoided official definitions and resisted the temptation to label individuals as poor. Yet the women in this study were poor and were very much aware that they were poor. As previously discussed, Oppenheim and Harker (1996) define poverty in a richer way than official statistics:

'Poverty means going short materially, socially and emotionally. It means spending less on food, on heating, and on clothing than someone on an average income. Above all, poverty takes away the tools to build the blocks for the future – your life chances. It steals away the opportunity to have a life unmarked by sickness, a decent education, a secure home and a long retirement' (1996:4).

For the women in this study, poverty seemed to limit their choices and options. To be poor and a woman limits choices even further. The universal solutions are determined by this predominant analysis of poverty. It is accepted that women living in poverty are disadvantaged in many ways; they are more likely to be ill and their children are more likely, to be ill or die at an early age. They are more likely to have a low birth-weight baby; the incidence is now 25 per cent higher for social classes IV and V than for others. Babies born to lone mothers are still more likely to have a low birth weight (ONS Children and Families Section 1998). As women in poverty, they are less likely to have a decent education and are denied the opportunities of employment as they care for small children. However, this is only one 'way of seeing'; it is a perception set in the context of my values, my belief systems. It is clear that some women will not suffer these disadvantages; they will continue to produce healthy babies, of normal weight, who remain well. Their chances of a decent education are noticeably less; having a baby at 15 years of age must be considered a disadvantage and steps should be taken to provide second-chance education. My interpretation was that the women in this study did indeed go short materially, socially and emotionally; most lived in what I regarded as poor-quality housing that was cold and in need of repair and maintenance. On a daily basis most coped with the drudgery and hardship of making ends meet; they managed the money, borrowed from Peter to pay Paul, and worked out how to survive until the next Giro cheque became due. As childbearing women, living in poverty, my respondents had limited economic, social and political power.

Childbearing and child rearing in combination with poverty rendered some of these women relatively powerless, socially excluded, stressed and denied the opportunities to become either educated or employed. For some, motherhood was seen as a certainty in their lives and having children was seen as negating some of the day-to-day negative effects of living in poverty. Some chose to have children as a means of finding pleasure and to give meaning to otherwise unhappy lives. Women's progress in the public sphere has been resisted for many centuries. As Rosalind Miles (1988) contends there has always been resentment against women who took men's jobs, left the isolation of the home and thus 'neglected' their children. They sought solidarity with other women, secured an income (even if the income was inadequate and derived from state benefits), learned to do 'masculine' things like decorating and sometimes left abusive relationships. The women in this study were no different: some had achieved some financial independence; they had built relationships with other women, mainly their mother; but they had difficulty in seeing the opportunities and advantages of paid employment or indeed education.

In chapter three, I described the research methodology. I have debated the use of interviews and challenged the notions of objectivity and truth. I have used qualitative research and, as such, it is both subjective and interpretative. It contains biases and values and reflects the choices that I made as the researcher. I chose which words to interpret and which themes to develop, and in so doing, I chose which aspects to ignore. My choices were influenced by my beliefs and values and by my knowledge and experiences; I established a relationship both with the respondents and with the subject matter. I was reflexive but my biases and beliefs may be buried too deeply to recognise. What Mauthner and Doucet (1998) refer to as the 'unconscious filters' through which we experience the world may be too difficult to uncover. I was also faced with what is a major dilemma of feminist qualitative research: making public, in the academic world, the private lives of a disadvantaged group.

I was allowed the privilege of sharing in the lives of a group of women who were disadvantaged by poverty. I was able to share in some aspects of their private lives and be party to some of their most intimate and emotional experiences. My task as an academic is to bring this intimate private world to the public world. It requires sensitivity, the ability to live with the discomfort of making public the private and a deeply held conviction that such exposure is justified. I believe that the work is important because it demonstrates the harsh reality of being a childbearing woman living in poverty at the end of the twentieth century and the messages for midwives and other health professionals are worth sharing. The publicly collected government statistics do not describe the private issues of those living in poverty nor the complexities of everyday life on state benefits, neither do they measure freedom or happiness.

In chapter four, I explored the concept of motherhood and further examined the shared themes of responsibility and respectability. I found that there were similarities amongst the differences in women. I found that, for some women, to be a 'good mother' was very important and brought satisfaction, respectability and a sense of personal worth. They shared a belief in putting their children's needs first and in many cases it was this belief that guided their actions.

In chapter five, I describe how different women with different experiences found different ways of managing their lives and surviving a life in poverty. Many of the women in this study had stable relationships and considerable support from their own mother rather than from their husbands or partners. It was women supporting women that dominated the patterns of relationships. The grandmothers were actively involved with child care and had a close relationship with their grandchildren, a fact supported by the British Social Attitudes Survey, published in December 1999 (Ezard 1999). The grandmothers helped with the domestic chores, shared the child-care responsibilities and were the source of company and emotional support. The men, without a job and without a commitment to a family, were marginalised, excluded and left to find a new purpose and identity. Men had to face bewildering changes in both their roles and their expectations; the traditional hierarchies associated with being a wage earner and provider for the family had disappeared. The men heard the women use the phrase '*no wage, no use*', and it was the men who were unable to do anything about their position. The violence that some women experienced could be explained, but not excused, by the frustrations of men with no sense of purpose or value in life. The latest statistics on young male suicides would seem to support a growing bafflement with their lives. Young men without a known occupation are nearly four times as vulnerable to suicide as those in social class I and II (Drever and Whitehead 1997a, 1997b).

In chapter six, I explored the changing nature of the relationships between childbearing women and the *restless men* in their lives. I found that individual women found different ways of resolving challenging relationships and how they exercised their knowledge and power to find solutions that were acceptable to them. As strong women, rather than powerless victims, some women had learned to fend for themselves and began to enjoy the peace of living alone. They found that they coped well without the support from the restless men in their lives. Their experiences and life styles were not unique: the *General Household Survey* published in December 1999 (ONS 1999) showed that one in four couples tried and failed to live together; 23 per cent of men and women aged 25-34 said they had previously cohabited with a partner without it leading to marriage (*Social Trends 31*, ONS 2001).

Many women learned to live with the horror of the crime of domestic violence and, in chapter seven, I have explored some women's experiences. Over half the sample of women were abused, but slightly less than half were not. I found that whilst domestic violence was a common experience, different women found different ways of surviving the violence. Some developed tactics to minimise the harm whilst others chose to live alone. In many cases, the women had quite limited choices; with very little money and dependent young children, they had nowhere to go and no means of going. Some endured and tolerated domestic violence; their options were limited by a lack of money and by a lack of material possessions; others stayed and put up with the injuries. Some had normalised violence which they took to be an everyday part of their lives.

In their childbearing experience, the women in this study also had to cope with the negative attitudes adopted by their carers. In chapter eight, I describe how some women felt that they were 'othered' and 'pathologised' by midwives and other health-care professionals. Many hospital-based midwives had negative attitudes to them simply because they were poor. They saw women through beliefs based on stereotypes and prejudice. It was clear that some hospital-based midwives needed to be better informed and to have the opportunity to understand some of the complexities of poverty. Birth should be a time of affirmation and negative comments made at this time can have a disproportionately damaging effect on women. Some midwives still need to recognise the effects and potential effects of poverty rather than blame the woman who is in some way the victim of that poverty. Some midwives still need to learn to recognise domestic violence and learn how to help and support women through the impossible choices they have to face. If anything, midwives have to recognise the power they have as professionals and the ability that comes with that power to abuse already disadvantaged women. Working in partnership with women means casting aside stereotypical views and judgemental attitudes. It means working alongside women, giving them time and human contact. It means that each midwifery meeting should be an opportunity for a human encounter and a real willingness to share and listen. It also means working closely with others: community leaders, other health professionals and the women who support the mothers. Most of all, midwives have to think more about their care and more about the ways in which they can enhance a woman's experience of childbirth and minimise the effects of poverty. Despite closer working between agencies, new partnerships, collaboration between health and social care providers, Health Improvement Programmes and a plethora of government initiatives, it was the attitudes of some midwives that shaped their childbearing experiences.

RECOMMENDATIONS FOR PRACTICE

Midwives working in the NHS today are part of a very structured organisation. In response to predominantly white middle-class criticism of maternity care, the maternity services have sought to become more consumer orientated. Great efforts have been made to improve the physical environment of maternity units. Wallpaper and potted plants have appeared in labour wards; midwives are organised into teams with the hope of providing greater continuity of care and carer. Women are encouraged to exercise choice over aspects of their childbirth experience and are handed out leaflets explaining the pros and cons of various options. Communication skills are taught as part of all midwifery education programmes. It is argued that midwifery is moving away from paternalistic care towards partnership and collaboration, the new buzzwords of the modernised NHS. Within this structural change, individual midwives are seeking to provide midwifery care to very different women from different backgrounds and with different experiences. The structures and policies of the maternity services and the NHS are at best broad-brush approaches to care. The needs of individuals are frequently lost in the organisation and the system. This research has demonstrated how the individual is also frequently lost within the system. When I spoke to the midwives who worked in Middleton and who knew the women and the community very well, they said that they had no idea that domestic violence was an issue nor had they any idea of what some women thought of the maternity care offered in the area. This study has already made a significant difference to some women in Middleton. Alongside a community midwife, I was able to persuade the health authority to fund a full-time midwife to work with other agencies to support pregnant women who faced domestic violence. This study could be criticised because it focuses on a small group of women, but it listened to their individual needs and, using political influences and structures, was able to make a difference. It is a 'microsociological' study; it focuses on the detail in the context of the 'macrosociological' or big picture.

It challenges midwives to understand and recognise the subjectivity of their own experiences.

It is important to summarise the lessons from this research and to offer some recommendations for practice. I consider that midwives in particular should think carefully about the clear messages from the women who contributed to this study. I believe that midwives should:

- Always be aware that not all women are the same and not all women on state benefits are the same.
- Recognise that women are different; they have different experiences, different backgrounds and different needs.
- Avoid making assumptions about any woman.
- Not assume that they understand women's needs and their problems by simply referring to their address or postal code or appearance.
- Not assume that women bringing up a family on state benefits are always hungry, in need of practical support and living in poor housing; they may be managing very well.
- Avoid giving blanket, impractical and unrealistic advice, especially about diet, smoking and other life-style choices. They should listen and respond to individuals.
- Avoid making judgements about how other people spend what money they have.
- Not assume that being poor means being of low intellect or stupid.
- Not assume that women living in poverty are always reluctant to be pregnant or assume they have made a wrong decision.
- Not assume that women have become pregnant to get a flat, a house or improve their benefit income.
- Not assume all women are happily married, heterosexual, have freedom to make choices and are automatically happy with their lot in life.
- Remember that what matters more to women is not so much being disadvantaged by poverty, 'race' or by disability but being disadvantaged by the attitudes and reactions of those involved in their care.
- Avoid becoming intolerant of those whose life styles and choices differ from their own.
- Remember that women from disadvantaged groups are human beings first, disadvantaged second.

And finally:

- Be willing to see the person, engage with women, give of themselves, make human contact, listen and wherever possible add a spiritual dimension to their care (see also Hunt 2001).

It is by attending to these issues that midwives can make a difference to the individual lives of women facing childbirth whilst living in poverty.

I also found very little evidence to confirm the findings of the *Changing Childbirth* report (DoH 1993). For the women in this study choice, control and continuity of carer were far less important to them than the negative attitudes adopted by some midwives. They told me that they wanted to be treated as individuals. Some women told me that for them it was not important that they knew the midwife who cared for them in labour; what was important was that she treated them with respect and was technically competent. They did value the relationship that they had with community midwives so perhaps continuity of carer was important to them in that setting. They did not feel choice was an issue; they were happy to follow the 'expert's' advice. They did not feel that control was an issue, but they desperately wanted to be treated with respect, be seen as 'respectable' and be seen as a good mother. They wanted the midwives to acknowledge that they were responsible parents who were making the most of their limited resources and were doing their best for their children.

As a result of my experiences undertaking this research, I believe that childbearing women living in poverty do not want sympathy or charity. They do need to be treated with dignity and respect and to be recognised as valuable and equal members of society. They also need government intervention and structural change. They need more money, that is certain, but they also need affordable, accessible child care so that they can exercise the choice to work and be economically independent. Some feel that they need the opportunity to gain educational qualifications and new skills if they are to earn enough to make coming off benefits worthwhile. Some feel that they need access to a refuge and the transport to get there if the violence in their life becomes intolerable. Some women feel that they need a second chance at education and training with the right physical and environmental support. The answer to poverty would be work, but only in these circumstances. Another structural change would be the abolition of fuel debt. In the same way that there has been a national campaign to wipe out Third World debt, there should be a similar campaign to abolish fuel debt. For poor families and the elderly, struggling to repay fuel debt out of an already inadequate income is impossible. The costs of wiping the slate clean would be minimal and would give poor people a real chance to get ahead. When up to one third of state benefits is withheld to repay fuel debt it is impossible for pregnant women to eat a reasonable diet and make ends meet. I am aware that these are, fundamentally, feminist solutions borne out of a desire to restore power to women. I do not believe that an acknowledgement of the poststructuralist nature of women mutually excludes the possibility of reforming structures to support the individual. The two can and should be compatible. Only by considering the two together are we likely to achieve any positive change. Structuralism and agency are not mutually exclusive; neither should be rejected in favour of the other.

CONCLUSIONS AND RECOMMENDATIONS FOR FURTHER RESEARCH

This study has been challenging, fascinating and sometimes frustrating. The lives of childbearing women living in poverty are complex, often contradictory and frequently intense. Their lives are dominated by the need to survive, to make ends meet and care for their children. Whilst there is overwhelming evidence of the link between poverty and ill health, many remained physically and emotionally well. They were strong women who were able to juggle the competing demands of poverty, pregnancy, small children and motherhood with the stresses and strains of relationships that were unsupportive and often in conflict. They were survivors who fight the system whether the 'system' is the state or the medical/midwifery professions. State benefits play a vital role in the survival of these women. The amount should be sufficient to ensure that no woman or her children lives below the poverty line. That is the least they should expect from a just and civilised society.

I believe that ethnographic research such as this is still one of the most effective ways of researching some women's lives. The women I met would not respond to postal surveys or telephone polls. The interviews were successful because I took time to listen to the women and formed a trusting relationship with them. It was important to be part of the culture and to spend time living and working in the area. Although I still believe that ethnography was the most suitable methodology, the method has limitations, not least that the time and personal costs are considerable. Large-scale surveys, clinical trials and experimental research seek answers that can be generalised to populations, but within such studies the individuals are lost and their needs overlooked.

In midwifery research, much more needs to done to explore the individual experience of pregnancy and poverty. There is still a belief that the needs of individuals can be met by floral curtains, new wallpaper, complex off-duty rotas and the handing out of leaflets advocating choice. In particular, it would be worth considering ways of helping midwives to look beyond the external cues and to see the woman as an individual rather than a condition, a postal address or a social class. The difference I have seen in the attitudes of hospital and community midwives towards women who live in poverty is another important area for further research. There is also a danger in defining midwives as a homogeneous group and ignoring the work that individual midwives do with individual women.

Motherhood is an important concept and its place in the lives of childbearing women living in poverty needs further research. The role of grandmothers in supporting women is also deserving of further study. It would be worth considering why some women are so deeply involved in their children's family and if some grandmothers resent the limits such involvement places on their freedom.

The long and short-term effects of poverty and social exclusion on populations are currently being investigated by many researchers and government agencies. It is less common to single out the effects on women and unusual to study the impact of poverty on individual lives. In this research, it is evident that the individual effects are diverse. Apart from the known physical effects on population groups, individual women deal with the stresses and strains of their life style in a variety of ways. The long-term effects of poverty on women's physical and mental health are also worthy of further detailed investigation.

It would be important to understand more about the nature of men's responses to fatherhood and to women. There is a need to learn more about how some men relate to some women and why some men are more able to live in harmony with some women than others are. It is worth investigating why some men are willing and able to share the complex task of parenting and others are not. These were clearly important challenges for the young men who were in and out of women's lives.

Another important area for further research is the experience of fatherhood and poverty. The restless men described in this study are restless for a range of diverse reasons. The changing economic scene has left many of them disillusioned and without a clear focus in their lives. I believe that there is a need to move beyond the radical feminists' anger about all men and their inadequacies. To assume that all men are violent, oppressive and even fundamentally evil is simply incorrect. However, it is important to consider why some men physically and psychologically abuse some women. I would be interested in interviewing violent men and attempting to analyse some men's feelings, particularly after they have attacked a woman. This may be an area for men to research other men. There is also a need, at a time when violence has reached epidemic proportions, to understand more about the experience and the effects of living with domestic violence on women and on their children who frequently witness the violence.

Despite the limitations of studying a small group of women in one location, this study has made an important contribution to existing knowledge of childbearing women living in poverty at the end of the twentieth century. It is a unique study. It has used ethnographic methods and has involved a prolonged period of fieldwork. Through the research, I have listened to women who are rarely heard. The study has not ignored state policy or structures but has considered the impact of such policies on individuals. Most importantly, this study gave some women the opportunity to define their health-care agenda rather than being mere recipients of policy changes. This study provides midwives and others with the evidence that they need to look beyond the physical effects of poverty, to avoid making assumptions and stereotyping based on postal address and to endeavour to see women as individuals. The themes of responsibility, respectability and motherhood are important in seeing the woman beyond the postal address and beyond external images of poverty. Behind the external signs I found women who struggled to be seen as respectable, who had a well-developed sense of responsibility towards their children and who frequently lived with violent partners. These aspects of women's lives were unexpected. The traditional views of lives in poverty tend to focus on the physical effects of hardship whilst the issues that appear to motivate some women are rarely heard. What these women appear to want more than anything is to be treated with respect and dignity; they want to be treated as human beings, as women who are pregnant, who are responsible mothers, who are entitled to the same care as other women. They want financial support from the state when they are unable to work; they want the men in their lives to take on the responsibilities of parenthood and not to abuse them physically or mentally. Midwives and other health professionals can do a great deal to change their own attitudes and the nature of their care. The state can do much to ensure full employment and better education.

Despite the length and breadth of the study there is so much more to learn and understand. Having been duped into believing that the 'truth' was out there and waiting to be found, I found the diversity of truth occasionally disconcerting. It would be comfortable to draw firm conclusions about women's experiences of childbearing and poverty and to offer neat, simple solutions but research and life are not that simple.

References

Abbot E, Bombas K 1942 Pamphlet for the Women's Freedom League. In: Timmins N 1996 The five giants: a biography of the welfare state. Fontana Press, London

Abraham H 2000 Women's Aid Federation fact sheet 2001. Available at website: http://www.womensaid.org.uk/dv (accessed 20/08/02)

Acheson D 1998 Independent inquiry into inequalities in health report. Chairman: Sir Donald Acheson. The Stationery Office, London

Ackers L, Abbott P 1996 Social policy for nurses and the caring professions. Open University Press, Buckingham

Agar M H 1986 Speaking of ethnography, vol. 2. Sage, Beverly Hills

Alcock P 1997 Understanding poverty, 2nd edn. Macmillan, Basingstoke

Amott T L 1990 Black women and AFDC: making entitlement out of necessity. In: Gordon L (ed) Women, the state and welfare. University of Wisconsin Press, Madison

Andrews B, Brown G W 1988 Marital violence in the community: a biographical approach. British Journal of Psychiatry 153: 305-312

Annandale E 1998 The sociology of health and medicine. A critical introduction. Polity Press, Oxford

Atkinson P 1990 The ethnographic imagination. Routledge, London

Atkinson P 1995 Medical talk and medical work. Sage, London

Audit Commission 1998 First class delivery: a national survey of women's views of maternity care. Audit Commission Publications, Oxford

Bakowski M, Murch M, Walker V 1983 Marital violence: the community response. Tavistock Publications, London

Batty D 2002 Social exclusion: the issue explained. Guardian 15 January: 7

Beasley C 1999 What is feminism? Sage, London

Berkman L F 1984 Assessing the physical health effects of social networks and social support. American Review of Public Health 5: 413-432

Bernhard L A 1984 Feminist research in nursing research [poster presentation]. The First International Congress on Women's Health Issues. Halifax, Nova Scotia

Beveridge B 1942 Social insurance and allied services. Cmnd. 6404. HMSO, London

Bewley S, Friend J, Mezey G (eds) 1997 Violence against women. Royal College Obstetricics and Gynaecology, London

Bick D E, MacArthur C 1995 The extent, severity and effect of health problems after childbirth. British Journal of Midwifery 3 (1): 27-31

Bjornberg U (ed) 1992 European parents in the 1990s: contradictions and comparisons. Transaction Publishers, New Brunswick and London

Blackburn C 1991 Poverty and health: working with families. Open University Press, Milton Keynes

Blair T 1998 The third way: new politics for the new century. The Fabian Society, London

Bloor M 1978 On the analysis of observational data: a discussion of the worth and uses of inductive techniques and respondents validation. Sociology 12 (3): 545-552

BMA 1998 Domestic violence. British Medical Association, London

Bohn D 1990 Domestic violence and pregnancy: implications for practice. Journal Nurse Midwifery 35 (2): 86-88

Booth C 1894 The aged poor: condition. Macmillan, London

Botting B 1997 Mortality in childhood. In: Drever F, Whitehead M (eds) Health inequalities. Office of National Statistics, London

Bowen C 1954 Return to laughter. Gollancz, London. Cited in: Hammersley M, Atkinson P A 1995 Ethnography principles in practice, 2nd edn. Routledge, London

Bowler I 1993 They're not the same as us: midwives' stereotypes of south asian descent patients. Sociology of Health and Illness 15 (2): 158-177

Bradshaw J, Kennedy S, Kilkey M et al 1996 The employment of lone parents: a comparison of policy in twenty countries. Family Policy Studies Centre, Joseph Rowntree Foundation, London

Bradshaw J, Millar J 1991 Lone parents in the UK. HMSO, London

Braidotti R 1991 Plenary address. Women's Studies Network annual conference, London

Brannen J, Moss P 1987 Dual earner households: women's financial contributions after the birth of the first child. In: Brannen J, Wilson G (eds) Give and take in families: studies in resource distribution. Allen and Unwin, London

Brannen J, Moss P 1991 Managing mothers: dual earner households after maternity leave. Macmillan, London

Browne A 1987 When battered women kill. Collier Macmillan, London

Brynner J, Ferri E, Shepherd P (eds) 1997 Twenty-somethings in the 1990s. Ashgate Publishing Ltd, London

Bryson V 1999 Feminist debates: issues of theory and political practice. Macmillan, London

Bunting J 1997 Morbidity and health related behaviours of adults – a review. In: Drever F, Whitehead M (eds) Health inequalities. Office of National Statistics, London

Burgess R (ed) 1980 Field research: a sourcebook and field manual. Allen and Unwin, London

Cahill M 1994 The new social policy. Blackwell, London

Charles N 2000 Feminism, the state and social policy. Macmillan, London

Cobb S 1976 Social support as a moderator of life stress. Psychosomatic Medicine 38 (5): 300-314

Collins P 1991 Black feminist thought. Routledge, London

Cook J, Watt S 1992 Racism, women and poverty. In: Glendinning C, Millar J (eds) Women and poverty in Britain: the 1990s. Harvester Wheatsheaf, Hemel Hempstead

Corcoran M, Duncan G J, Hill M S 1986 The economic fortunes of women and children: lessons from the panel study of income dynamics. In: Gelphi B, Hartsock N C M, Novak C C et al (eds) Women and poverty. Chicago Press, Chicago

Cornwall J 1984 Hard-earned lives. Accounts of health and illness from East London. Tavistock Publications, London

Cragg A, Dawson T 1984 Unemployed women: a case study of attitudes and experiences. Department of Employment, London

Dahl T S 1987 Women's law: an introduction to feminist jurisprudence. Norwegian University Press, Oslo

Darling A 1999 Talking poverty. Guardian 8 December

Delamont S 1980 Sociology of women. George Allen and Unwin, London

Denzin N K (ed) 1970 Sociological methods: a source book. Butterworth, London

Department of Health 1993 Changing childbirth: Part 1 The report of the expert advisory group. HMSO, London

Department of Health 1996 On the state of the public health. The annual report of the Chief Medical Officer of the Department of Health for the year 1995. HMSO, London

Department of Health 1997 On the state of the public health. The annual report of the Chief Medical Officer of the Department of Health for the year 1996. HMSO, London

Department of Health 1998a The new NHS: modern, dependable. The Stationery Office, London

Department of Health 1998b Our healthier nation: a contract for health. The Stationery Office, London

Department of Health 1999 Saving lives: our healthier nation. The Stationery Office, London

Department of Health, Welsh Office, Scottish Office DoH, DoH and SS Northern Ireland 1998 Why mothers die: report on confidential enquiries into maternal deaths in the United Kingdom 1994-1996. The Stationery Office, London

Department of Health 2000 The NHS plan. http://www.doh.gov.uk/nhsplan/index

Department of Health and Social Services 1997 Well into 1997: a positive agenda for health and wellbeing. The Stationery Office, Belfast

Department of Health, Welsh Office, Scottish Office DoH, DoH and SS Northern Ireland 2001 Why mothers die: report on confidential enquiries into maternal deaths in the United Kingdom 1997-1999. The Stationery Office, London

Department of Social Security 1994 Households below average income 1979-1991/92: a statistical analysis. Government Statistical Service, HMSO, London

Department of Social Security 1998 Households below average income: 1979-1994/95. Government Statistical Service, HMSO, London

Dobash R E, Dobash R P 1977 Wives: the appropriate victims of marital violence. Victimology 2: 426-442

Dobson B, Beardsworth A, Keil T et al 1994 Diet, choice and poverty: social, cultural and nutritional aspects of food consumption among low income families. Family Policy Studies Centre, Loughborough University of Technology, Centre for Research in Social Policy, Loughborough

Donnison D 1998 Policies for a just society. Macmillan, Basingstoke

Dorling D 1999 The widening gap. 'Ministers fail to tackle biggest health gap'. Guardian 2 December: 6

Douglas J D 1985 Creative interviewing. Sage, Beverly Hills

Dowler E, Calvert C 1995 Nutrition and diet in lone-parent families in London. Family Policy Studies Centre supported by Joseph Rowntree Foundation, London

Doyal W, Wynn A, Wynn S et al 1991 Low birth weight and maternal diet. Midwife Health Visitor and Community Nurse 27: 44-45

Drever F, Whitehead M 1997a Health inequalities. Office of National Statistics, London

Drever F, Whitehead M 1997b Health inequalities. Decennial supplement [dataset]. Office of National Statistics, London

Dunn H G 1984 Social aspects of low birth weight. Canadian Medical Association Journal 130: 1131-1140

Durkin T 1997 Using computers in strategic qualitative research. In: Millar G, Dingwall R (eds) Context and method in qualitative research. Sage, London

Edgell S 1993 Class. Routledge, London

Elias P 1997 Social class and the standard occupational classification. In: Rose D, O'Reilly K (eds) Constructing classes: towards a new social classification for the UK. ESRC/Office of National Statistics, Swindon

Ezard J 1999 Grannies regain key role in family life. Guardian 1 December: 3

Fall C H D, Vijayamukar M, Barker D J P et al 1995 Weight in infancy and prevalence of coronary heart disease in adult life. British Medical Journal 310: 17-19

Ferri E, Smith K 1996 Parenting in the 1990s. Family Policy Studies Centre supported by Joseph Rowntree Foundation, London

Field F 1989 Losing out: the emergence of Britain's underclass. Blackwell, London

Forsen T, Eriksson J, Tuomilehto J et al 1997 Mother's weight in pregnancy and coronary heart disease in a cohort of Finnish men: follow-up study. British Medical Journal 315: 837-840

Foucault M 1980 Power/knowledge: selected interviews and other writings. Penguin, Harmondsworth

Foucault M 1983 The subject and power [trans Sawyer]. In: Dreyfus H L, Rainbow P (eds) Michel Foucault: Beyond structuralism and hermeneutics. University of Chicago Press, Chicago

Francis B 1999 Modernist reductionism or post-structuralist relativism: can we move on? An evaluation of the arguments in relation to feminist educational research. Gender and Education 11 (4): 381-393

Furstenburg F 1992 Teenage childbearing and cultural rationality: a thesis in search of evidence. Family Relations 41 (2): 244-248

Gayford J J 1978 Battered wives. In: Martin J P (ed) Violence and the family. John Wiley and Sons, New York

George V, Howards I 1991 Poverty amidst affluence: Britain and the United States. Edward Elgar, London

Giddens A 1984 The constitution of society. Polity Press, Cambridge

Giddens A 1993 Sociology, 2nd edn. Polity Press, Cambridge

Giddens A 1999 Is there such a thing as the third way? Guardian 23 May

Glendinning C, Millar J (eds) 1992 Women and poverty in Britain in the 1990s. Harvester Wheatsheaf, London

Gowridge C, Williams A S, Wynn M (eds) 1997 Mother courage: letters from mothers in poverty at the end of the century. Penguin Books, London

Graham H 1984 Women, health and the family. Wheatsheaf Books, London

Graham H 1987a Being poor: perceptions and coping strategies of lone mothers. In: Brannen J, Wilson G (eds) Give and take in families: studies in resource distribution. Allen and Unwin, London

Graham H 1987b Women's smoking and family health. Social Science and Medicine 25 (1): 47-56

Graham H 1993 Women's smoking: government targets and social trends. Health Visitor 66 (3)

Graham H 1998 Health inequalities and the public health green papers. Health Variations 2, July

Green D G 1998 Benefit dependency. How welfare undermines independence. Choices in Welfare 41. The Institute of Economic Affairs Health and Welfare Unit, London

Grieve Smith J 1999 Welfare weasels. Guardian 2 December: 6

Guardian 1988 [leader]. Guardian 23 November

Guardian 2002 The class war is over [leader]. Guardian 22 August: 8

Hales C N, Barker D J P, Clark P M S et al 1991 Fetal and infant growth and impaired glucose tolerance at age 64. British Medical Journal 303: 1019-1022

Hammersley M, Atkinson P A 1995 Ethnography principles in practice, 2nd edn. Routledge, London

Hantrais L 1995 Social policy in Europe. Routledge, London

Harding S (ed) 1987 Feminism and methodology: social science issues. Indiana University Press, Bloomington

Harding S 1991 Feminism and theories of scientific knowledge. In: Evans M (ed) The woman question, 2nd edn 1994. Sage, London

Harding S 1993 Rethinking standpoint epistemology: what is 'strong objectivity'? In: Alcoff L, Potter E (eds) Feminist epistemologies. Routledge, New York

Hart A, Lockey R, Henwood F et al 2001 Addressing inequalities in health: new directions in midwifery education and practice. English National Board for Nursing, Midwifery and Health Visiting, London

Hart J T 1971 The inverse care law. Lancet: 405-412

Hawkesworth M E 1989 Knowers, knowing, known: feminist theory and claims of truth. SIGNS: Journal of Women in Culture and Society 14 (3): 533-557

Hays S 1996 The cultural contradictions of motherhood. Yale University Press, London

Helton A S, Anderson E, McFarlane J 1987 Battered and pregnant: a prevalence study with intervention measures. American Journal of Public Health 77: 1337-1339

Hester M, Kelly L, Radford J (eds) 1996 Women, violence and male power. Open University Press, Buckingham

Hillard P A 1985 Physical abuse in pregnancy. Obstetrics and Gynaecology 66: 185-190

Hills J 1996 New inequalities the changing distribution of income and wealth in the United Kingdom. Cambridge University Press, Cambridge

Hobbs D, May T 1993 Interpreting the field accounts of ethnography. Clarendon Press, Oxford

Hobson B 1990 No exit, no voice: women's economic dependency and the welfare state. Acta Sociologica 33 (3): 235-250

Holland J, Ramazanoğlu C 1994 Coming to conclusions: power and interpretation in researching young women's sexuality. In: Maynard M, Purvis J (eds) Researching women's lives from a feminist perspective. Taylor and Francis, London

Holman R 1978 Poverty: explanations of social deprivation. Martin Robertson, London

Holmes T H, Rae R H 1967 Social readjustment rating scale. Journal of Psychosomatic Research 11: 219-224

Holstein J, Gubrium J F 1998 Active interviewing. In: Silverman D (ed) Qualitative research theory, method and practice. Sage, London

Holton R, Turner B 1994 Debate and pseudo-debate in class analysis: some unpromising aspects of Goldthorpe and Marshall's defense. Sociology 28 (3): 799-804

Home Office 1993 Domestic violence review. Report of the select committee on domestic violence. HMSO, London

Home Office 2001 Criminal statistics in England and Wales 2000. HMSO, London

Howarth C, Kenway P, Palmer G et al 1998 Monitoring poverty and social exclusion. Labour's inheritance. New Policy Institute and Joseph Rowntree Foundation, London

Howe G, Westhoff C, Vesset M et al 1985 Effects of age, cigarette smoking and other factors on fertility. British Medical Journal 290: 1697

Hughes J A, Sharrock W W 1997 The philosophy of social research, 3rd edn. Longmans Higher Education, London

Humphreys J 1993 Children of battered women. In: Campbell J C, Humphreys J (eds) Nursing care of survivors of family violence. Mosby, St Louis

Hunt S C 2001 Tackling disadvantage in maternity care. In: Midwives in action: a resource. English National Board for Nursing, Midwifery and Health Visiting, London

Hunt S C, Martin A M 2001 Pregnant women, violent men: what midwives need to know. Butterworth Heinemann, Oxford

Hunt S C, Symonds A 1995 The social meaning of midwifery. Macmillan, Basingstoke

Hyndman S J 1990 Housing damp and health among British Bengalis in East London. Social Science and Medicine 30: 131-141

Jay, Baroness of Paddington 1999 Listening to women [letter]. Guardian 8 December: 23

Jowell R, Witherspoon S, Brook L et al 1990 British social attitudes: the 7th report. Gower, Aldershot

Kahn R, Antonucci T 1980 Convoys over the life course: attachment, roles and social support. In: Baltes P B, Brim O (eds) Life-span development and behaviour. Lexington Press, Boston

Kaplan E A 1992 Motherhood and representation. Routledge, London

Kiernan K E, Estaugh V 1993 Cohabitation extra-marital childbearing and social policy. Family Policy Studies Centre/Joseph Rowntree Foundation, London

Kirk J, Miller M L 1986 Reliability and validity in qualitative research. Sage, London

Kirkwood C 1993 Leaving abusive partners. Sage, London.

Kroll D (ed) 1996 Midwifery care for the future. Ballière Tindall, London

Lareau A, Shultz J 1996 Journeys through ethnography. Realistic accounts of fieldwork. Westview Press

Lash S, Urry J 1996 Economies of signs and space. Sage Publications, London

LeCompte M D, Goetz J P 1982 Problems of reliability and validity in ethnographic research. Review of Educational Research 52: 31-60

Leiberman E 1995 Low birth weight – not a black and white issue. New England Journal of Medicine 332: 117-118

Leininger M M 1985 Ethnography and ethno-nursing: models and modes of qualitative data analysis. In: Leininger M M (ed) Qualitative research methods in nursing. Grune and Stratton Inc, Orlando

Lewis G 2001 Domestic violence. In: Department of Health, Welsh Office, Scottish Office DoH, DoH and SS Northern Ireland 1999 Why mothers die: report on confidential enquiries into maternal deaths in the United Kingdom 1997-1999. The Stationery Office, London

Lewis J, Piachaud D 1992 Women and poverty in the twentieth century. In: Glendinning C, Millar J (eds) Women and poverty in Britain in the 1990s. Harvester Wheatsheaf, London

Lewis O 1965 The children of Sanchez. Penguin, London

Lewis O 1966 The culture of poverty. Scientific American 215, October

Lewis O 1968 La vida. Panther, London

Lincoln Y, Guba E 1985 Naturalistic enquiry. Sage, Newbury Park

Lister R 1997 Citizenship. Feminist perspectives. Macmillan, Basingstoke

Lister R 1999 Building an inclusive society. Annual lecture on social change, Birmingham, 8 June; also in Guardian 9 June: Society 6

Lofland J, Lofland L H 1984/1995 Analysing social settings: a guide to qualitative observation and analysis, 2nd edn. Wadsworth, Belmont

Lonsdale S 1990 Women and disability. Macmillan, Basingstoke

Lovenduski J, Randall V 1993 Contemporary feminist politics: women and power. Oxford University Press, Oxford

MacArthur C, Lewis M, Knox E G 1991 Health after childbirth. HMSO, London

Mack J, Lansley S 1985 Poor Britain. Allen and Unwin, London

Mack J, Lansley S 1992 Breadline Britain 1990s, the findings of the television series. London Weekend Television, London

Marshall T H 1950 Citizenship and social class and other essays. In: Charles N 2000 Feminism, the state and social policy. Macmillan, Basingstoke

Maternity Alliance 1995 Poor expectations: poverty and under-nourishment in pregnancy. Maternity Alliance, London

Mauthner N, Doucet A 1998 Reflections on a voice-centred relational method. In: Ribbens J, Edwards R (eds) Feminist dilemmas in qualitative research. Public knowledge and private lives. Sage Publications, London

Mayall B, Hood S, Oliver S 1999 Introduction. In: Hood S, Mayall B, Oliver S (eds) Critical issues in social research power and prejudice. Open University Press, Buckingham

Mayo M, Weir A 1993 The future for feminist social policy. In: Page R, Baldock J (eds) Social Policy Review 5: 35-57

McLaughlin E 1991 Social security and community care: the case of the invalid care allowance. Department of Social Security/HMSO, London

McMahon M 1995 Engendering motherhood: identity and self-transformation in women's lives. Guilford, New York

Mezey G C 1997 Domestic violence and pregnancy. In: Bewley S, Friend J, Mezey G (eds) Violence against women. Royal College Obstetrics and Gynaecology, London

Mezey G C, Bewley S 1997a Domestic violence and pregnancy. British Journal of Obstetrics and Gynaecology 104: 528-531

Mezey G C, Bewley S 1997b Domestic violence in pregnancy. British Medical Journal 314, May

Miles I, Irvine J 1979 The critique of official statistics. In: Irvine J, Miles I, Evans J (eds) Demystifying statistics. Pluto, London

Miles M B, Huberman A M 1994 Qualitative data analysis, 2nd edn. Sage, London

Miles R 1988 The woman's history of the world. Paladin, London

Milham S, Davis R L 1991 Cigarette smoking during pregnancy and mother's occupation. Journal of Occupational Medicine 33: 468-473

Millar J 1989 Poverty and the lone parent: the challenge to social policy. Averbury, Aldershot

Miller J, Glassner B 1998 The 'inside' and the 'outside': finding realities in interviews. In: Silverman D (ed) Qualitative research theory, method and practice. Sage, London

Mooney J 1993 The hidden figure: the north London domestic violence survey. University Centre for Criminology, London

Morse J M, Field P A 1996 Nursing research. the application of qualitative approaches, 2nd edn. Chapman Hall, London

Murcott A (ed) 1998 The nation's diet: the social science of food choice. Addison Wesley Longman, London

Murray C 1990 The emerging British underclass. IEA Health and Welfare Unit, London

Murray C 1994 Underclass: the crisis deepens. IEA Health and Welfare Unit, London

Mutale T, Creed F, Maresh M et al 1991 Life events and low birth weight: analyses by infant preterm and small for gestational age. British Journal of Obstetrics and Gynaecology 98: 166-172

Navarro V 1994 The politics of health policy: the US reforms 1980-1994. Blackwell, Oxford

Nichols T 1979 Social class: official, sociological and Marxist. In: Irvine J, Miles I, Evans J (eds) Demystifying social statistics. Pluto, London

Oakley A 1974 The sociology of housework. Martin Robertson, Oxford

Oakley A 1979 From here to maternity: becoming a mother. Penguin, Harmondsworth

Oakley A 1992 Social support and motherhood. Blackwell, Oxford

Oakley A 1995 Interviewing women. In: Roberts H (ed) Doing feminist research. Routledge and Kegan Paul, London

Oakley A 1999 People's ways of knowing: gender and methodology. In: Hood S, Mayall B, Oliver S (eds) Critical issues in social research. Open University Press, Buckingham

O'Brian M 1981 The politics of reproduction. In: Barrett M et al (eds) Ideology and cultural production. Croom Helm, London

O'Brian M, Penna S 1998 Theorising welfare. Enlightenment and modern society. Sage, London

Office of National Statistics 1996/97 Family resources survey. The Stationery Office, London

Office of National Statistics 1997 General household survey. The Stationery Office, London

Office of National Statistics 1998a Labour force survey. Quarterly supplement. The Stationery Office, London

Office of National Statistics 1998b Social Trends 28. The Stationery Office, London

Office of National Statistics 1999 The general household survey. The Stationery Office, London

Office of National Statistics 2001 Social Trends 31. The Stationery Office, London

Office of National Statistics 2002 Social Trends 32. The Stationery Office, London

Office of National Statistics Children and Families Section 1998 Population and Health Monitor FMI 98/1. The Stationery Office, London

Office of National Statistics Monitor 1996 Population and Health DH3 96/3 no. 28. Infant and perinatal mortality – social and biological factors. Table 20, Table 4. DH3 97/2 Sudden infant deaths 1992-1996 Table 10. The Stationery Office, London

Office of National Statistics Monitor 2001 Population and Health DH3 no. 33 2001. Live births, still births and linked infant deaths: age of mother, inside marriage and outside marriage/joint registration by social class of father as defined by occupation, numbers and rates 2000 Table 20. The Stationery Office, London

O'Leary C M 1997 Counteridentification or counterhegemony? Transforming feminist standpoint theory. In: Kenney S J, Kinsella H (eds) Politics and feminist standpoint theories. Haworth, New York

Olesen V L 2000 Feminisms and qualitative research at and into the Millennium. In: Denzin N K, Lincoln Y S (eds) Handbook of qualitative research, 2nd edn. Sage, London

Olesen V L, Clarke A E 1999 Resisting closure, embracing uncertainties, creating agendas. In: Clarke A E, Olesen V L (eds) Revisioning women, health and healing: feminist, cultural and technoscience perspectives. Routledge, New York

Ong A 1995 Women out of China: travelling tales and travelling theories in postcolonial feminism. In: Behar R, Gordon D A (eds) Women writing culture. University of California Press, Berkeley

OPCS 1990 Infant feeding. Office of Population Censuses and Surveys. The Stationery Office, London

OPCS 1994 Social Trends 1994, no. 24, and 1995, no. 25. Office of Population Censuses and Surveys. The Stationery Office, London

OPCS 1995a Infant and perinatal mortality. Social and biological factors. Monitor DH3 95/3 no. 26, December. Office of Population Censuses and Surveys. The Stationery Office, London

OPCS 1995b Occupational health: Decennial supplement DS no. 10 (ed Drever F). Office of Population Censuses and Surveys/HMSO, London

Oppenheim C, Harker L 1996 Poverty: the facts, revised and updated, 3rd edn. Child Poverty Action Group, London

Orr J 1997 Nursing the academy. In: Stanley L (ed) Knowing feminisms. Sage Publications, London

Page L A (ed) 2000 The new midwifery: science and sensitivity in practice. Churchill Livingston, Edinburgh and London

Pahl J 1989 Money and marriage. Macmillan, London

Parsons M 1998 200 years from poverty to decency. A review of social conditions from laissez-faire to Fabian socialism and back. Available at: http://www.users.on.net/rmc/200yspt (accessed 16/11/98)

Payne S 1991 Women, health and poverty: an introduction. Harvester Wheatsheaf, London

Pember Reeves M 1911 Round about a pound a week. Virago, London

Perakyla A 1998 Reliability and validity in research based on tapes and transcripts. In: Silverman D (ed) Qualitative research theory, method and practice. Sage, London

Phoenix A 1991 Young mothers? Polity Press, Cambridge

Phillimore P 1989 Shortened lives: premature death in North Tyneside. Bristol Papers in Applied Social Studies 12. University of Bristol, Bristol

Piachaud D 1981 Peter Townsend and the Holy Grail. New Society 10 September

Piachaud D 1987a Poverty in Britain 1899 to 1983. Journal of Social Policy 17 (3): 335-351

Piachaud D 1987b Problems in the definition and measurement of poverty. Journal of Social Policy 16 (10): 226-238

Prescott-Clarke P, Primatesta P 1998 Health survey for England 1996. The Stationery Office, London

Radford L, Hester M, Pearson C 1998 Domestic violence fact sheet. Women's Aid Federation, Bristol

Rahman M, Palmer G, Kenway P 2001 Monitoring poverty and social exclusion 2001. New Policy Institute/Joseph Rowntree Foundation, York

Ramazanoğlu C (ed) 1993 Up against Foucault: explorations of some tensions between Foucault and feminism. Routledge, London

Ramsay J, Richardson J, Carter Y H et al 2002 Should health professionals screen women for domestic violence? Systematic review. British Medical Journal 325: 326

Rex J 1973 Race, colonialism and the city. Routledge and Kegan Paul, London

Ribbens J, Edwards R (eds) 1998 Feminist dilemmas in qualitative research. Public knowledge and private lives. Sage Publications, London

Richardson L 1993 The case of the skipped line: poetics, dramatics and transgressive validity. Sociological Quarterly

Roberts D E 1995 Race, gender and the value of mother's work. Social Politics 2 (2): 195-207

Roll J 1992 Understanding poverty. A guide to the concepts and measures. Family Policy Studies Centre, London

Rose D, O'Reilly K 1998 Constructing classes: toward a new social classification for the UK. ESRC/ONS, Swindon

Roseneil S 1993 Greenham revisited: researching myself and my sisters. In: Hobbs D, May T (eds) Interpreting the field. Clarendon Press, Oxford

Rothwell H 1995 The diets of pregnant women dependent on low incomes [unpublished BSc midwifery thesis]. University of Wales College of Medicine, Cardiff

Rowbotham S 1974 Hidden from history, 2nd edn. Pluto Press, London

Rowntree B S 1941 Poverty and progress: a second social survey of York. Longman,London

Rowntree B, Lavers G 1951 Poverty and the welfare state. Longman, London

Rowntree B, Seebohm M 1901 Poverty: a study of town life. Macmillan, London

Royal College of Obstetrics and Gynaecology 2001 Why mothers die 1997-1991: the confidential enquiries into maternal deaths in the United Kingdom. RCOG Press, London

Runciman W G 1990 How many classes are there in British society? Sociology 24: 378-396

Rutter D R, Quine L 1990 Inequalities in pregnancy outcome: a review of psychosocial and behavioural mediators. Social Science Medicine 30: 553-568

Sandelowski M 1986 The problem of rigour in qualitative research. Advances in Nursing Science 8: 27-37

Sandelowski M 1993 Rigour or rigor mortis: the problems of rigour in qualitative research revisited. Advances in Nursing Science 16 (2): 1-8

Schaefer C, Coyne J C, Lazarus R S 1981 The health-related functions of social support. Journal of Behavioural Medicine 4 (4): 381-405

Scheper-Hughes N 1992 Death without weeping: the violence of everyday life in Brazil. University of California Press, Berkeley

Sexton M, Hebel J R 1984 A clinical trial of change in maternal smoking and its effect on birth weight. Journal of American Medical Association 251: 911-915

Silverman D 1993 Interpreting qualitative data methods for analysing talk, text and interaction. Sage Publications, London

Silverman D (ed) 1998 Qualitative research theory, method and practice. Sage, London

Skeggs B 1997 Formations of class and gender. Sage, London

Smith L 1989 Domestic violence. HMSO, London

Spelman E V 1988 Inessential woman. Problems of exclusion in feminist thought. Beacon Press, Boston

Spradley J P 1979 The ethnographic interview. Holt, Reinhart and Winston, New York

Spradley J P 1980 Participant observation. Holt, Reinhart and Winston, New York

Stacey J 1988 Can there be a feminist ethnography? Women's Studies International Forum 11 (1): 21-27

Stacey J 1997 Feminist theory: capital F, capital T. In: Robinson V, Richardson D (eds) Introducing women's studies, 2nd edn. Macmillan, Basingstoke

Stanley L 1985 Biography as microscope or kaleidoscope. In: Farren D et al (eds) Writing feminist biography. Studies in Sexual Politics 13/14. University of Manchester, Manchester

Stark E, Flitcraft A 1996 Women at risk. Sage, London

Strachan D 1986 The home environment and respiratory morbidity in children. Paper presented at the Conference of Unhealthy Housing, University of Warwick.

Symonds A, Hunt S C 1996 The midwife and society. Perspectives, policies and practice. Macmillan, Basingstoke

Taylor-Gooby P 1990 Social welfare, the unkindest cut of all. In: Jowell R (ed) British social attitudes. The seventh report, social and community planning research. Gower, Aldershot

Taylor-Gooby P, Dale J 1981 Social theory and social welfare. Arnold, London

Thomas R 1990 Occupation referenced socio economic classification. Survey Methodology Bulletin 26: 26-34

Timmins N 1996 The five giants: a biography of the welfare state. Fontana Press, London

Townsend P 1979 Poverty in the UK. Penguin, Harmondsworth

Townsend P 1993 Underclass and overclass: the widening gulf between social classes in Britain in the 1980s. In: Payne G, Cross M (eds) Sociology in action. Macmillan, London

Townsend P 1995 The rise of international social policy. The Policy Press, Brighton

Townsend P, Davidson N 1982 The Black report. Inequalities in health (reprint 1986). Penguin: Harmondsworth

Toynbee P 1999 This is what women want. Guardian 18 June: 19

UNDP 1996 Human development report. Oxford University Press, Oxford and New York. Available at: http://www.user.on.net/hdro,undp (accessed 11/11/98)

Venanzi A 2000 The concept of exclusion. Available at: http://www.mailbase.ac.uk/lists-p-t/social-theory/1998-05/0027.html (accessed 06/05/00)

Vogel J, Anderssen L G, Davidson U et al 1988 Inequality in Sweden: trends and current situation. SCB, Stockholm

Walby S 1997 Gender transformations. Routledge, London

Waldmann R J 1992 Income distribution and infant mortality. Quarterly Journal of Economics 107: 1283-1302. Cited in: Wilkinson R G 1996 Unhealthy societies. Routledge, London

Walker D 2002 Poor deal. Guardian 11 April: 6

Walker L 1979 The battered woman. Harper and Row, New York

Walker L 1984 The battered women's syndrome. Springer, New York.

Walker R 1987 Consensual approaches to the definition of poverty. Journal of Social Policy 6: 7

Walsall Council Benefit Service/Benefit Agency Report 1998. Walsall MBC, Walsall

Walsall Health Authority 1997/8 Walsall public health report 1996. Walsall Health Authority, Walsall

Walsall Metropolitan Borough Council 1998 Annual employment survey. Walsall MBC, Walsall

Webb S 1993 Women's incomes: past, present and prospects. Fiscal Studies 14 (4): 14-36

Wedderburn D 1974 Poverty, inequality and class structure. Cambridge University Press, Cambridge

Weedon C 2000 Feminist practice and poststructuralist theory, 2nd edn. Blackwell, Oxford

West Midlands Regional Health Authority 1996 West Midlands life style survey. West Midlands Regional Health Authority, Birmingham

Whitehead M 1988 The health divide. Penguin, London

Wilkinson R G 1996 Unhealthy societies. Routledge, London

Wilkinson S (ed) 1986 Feminist social psychology: developing theory and practice. Open University Press, Milton Keynes

Wise S 1987 A framework for discussing ethical issues in feminist research: a review of the literature. In: Griffiths V, Humm M, O'Rourke R et al (eds) Writing feminist biography using life histories. Studies in Sexual Politics no. 19. Department of Sociology, University of Manchester, Manchester

Wolcott M 1992 Posturing in qualitative enquiry. In: LeCompte M, Millroy W L, Preissle J (eds) Handbook of qualitative research in education. California Academic Press, San Diego

Woolf V 1929/1994 A room of one's own. First published 1929, Great Britain: The Hogath Press; 1994 edn, Flamingo Modern Classics, London

World Health Organisation 1991 A strategy for health for all: revised targets. World Health Organisation, Copenhagen

Wynn S W, Wynn A H, Doyle W et al 1994 The association of maternal social class with maternal diet and dimensions of babies in a population of London women. Nutrition and Health 9 (4): 303-315

Zopf P 1989 American women in poverty. Grenwood Press, New York

Index